Anesthesia
for
Organ Transplantation

Edited by

Judith A. Fabian, MD

Associate Professor
Director, Cardiac Anesthesia
Medical College of Virginia
Richmond, VA

With additional 20 contributors

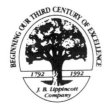

J. B. LIPPINCOTT COMPANY
Philadelphia

Anesthesia for Organ Transplantation

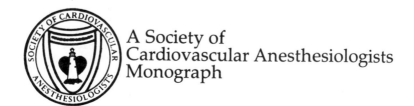

A Society of
Cardiovascular Anesthesiologists
Monograph

Acquisitions Editor: Mary K. Smith
Sponsoring Editor: Anne Geyer
Cover Designer: Anne O'Donnell
Production Manager: Robert D. Bartleson
Production Services: Nan Nagy
Compositor: University Graphics
Printer/Binder: R. R. Donnelly & Sons Company

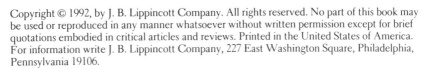

6 5 4 3 2 1

Library of Congress Cataloging in Publications Data

Anesthesia for organ transplantation / edited by Judith A. Fabian ;
   with 20 contributors.
      p.   cm.—(A Society of Cardiovascular Anesthesiologists
monograph)
    Includes index.
    ISBN 0-397-51172-8
    1. Heart—Transplantation. 2. Lungs—Transplantation. 3. Liver—
Transplantation. 4. Anesthesia. I. Fabian, Judith A.
II. Series.
    [DNLM: 1. Anesthesia, General—methods. 2. Organ Transplantation.
WO 660 A5796]
RD87.3.T7A547   1992
617.9'6795—dc20
DNLM/DLC
for Library of Congress   91-47980
                                                 CIP

The authors and publisher have exerted every effort to ensure that drug selection and dosage set forth in this text are in accord with current recommendations and practice at the time of publication. However, in view of ongoing research, changes in government regulations, and the constant flow of information relating to drug therapy and drug reactions, the reader is urged to check the package insert for each drug for any change in indications and dosage and for added warnings and precautions. This is particularly important when the recommended agent is a new or infrequently employed drug.

Publication Committee of the
Society of Cardiovascular Anesthesiologists

Contributors

Martin W. Allard, MB ChB, FFARCS
Associate Professor of Anesthesiology
Attending Anesthesiologist
Loma Linda University Medical
  Center
Loma Linda, California

The Reverend Roger A. Balk,
  PhD
Centre for Clinical Immunobiology
  and Transplantation
Royal Victoria Hospital
Transplant Service
Montreal, Quebec
Canada

Joel J. Berberich, MD, PhD
Associate Professor
Jefferson Medical College
Associate
Geisinger Medical Center
Danville, Pennsylvania

Carol M. Buchter, MD
Assistant Professor of Medicine
Case Western Reserve University
  School of Medicine
Staff Cardiologist
University Hospitals of Cleveland
Cleveland, Ohio

Verdi J. DiSesa, MD
Associate Professor of Surgery
University of Pennsylvania
Director of Cardiac Transplantation
Hospital of the University of
  Pennsylvania
Philadelphia, Pennsylvania

Cornelius M. Dyke, MD
Medical College of Virginia
McGuire VA Medical Center
Richmond, Virginia

Judith A. Fabian, MD
Associate Professor
Director, Cardiac Anesthesia
Medical College of Virginia
Richmond, Virginia

Simon Gelman, MD, PhD
Professor and Chairman
Department of Anesthesiology
Professor of Biology and Physiology
University of Alabama, Birmingham
The University Hospital
Birmingham, Alabama

Frederick A. Hensley, Jr., MD
Associate Professor of Anesthesia
The Pennsylvania State University
Director of Cardiac Anesthesia
University Hospital
The Milton S. Hershey Medical
    Center
Hershey, Pennsylvania

Kane M. High, MD
Assistant Professor of Anesthesia
The Pennsylvania State University
University Hospital
The Milton S. Hershey Medical
    Center
Hershey, Pennsylvania

Yoo Goo Kang, MD
Associate Professor
Department of Anesthesiology
University of Pittsburgh
Director, Hepatic Transplantation
    Anesthesiology
Presbyterian University Hospital
Pittsburgh, Pennsylvania

Loma Linda Pediatric Heart
    Group
Loma Linda University Medical
    Center
Loma Linda, California

Robert D. Martin, MD
Associate Professor of Anesthesiology
Attending Anesthesiologist
Loma Linda University Medical
    Center
Loma Linda, California

Harry I. McCarthy, II
Clinical Perfusionist
Medical College of Virginia
Richmond, Virginia

Jemi Olak, MSc, MD
Assistant Professor of Surgery
Division of Cardiothoracic Surgery
Medical College of Virginia
Medical College of Virginia Hospitals
Richmond, Virginia

Walter E. Pae, Jr., MD
Associate Professor of Surgery
The Pennsylvania State University
University Hospital
The Milton S. Hershey Medical
    Center
Hershey, Pennsylvania

G. Alexander Patterson, MD,
    FRCS (C) FACS
Professor of Surgery
Division of Cardiothoracic Surgery
Attending Physician
Barnes Hospital
St. Louis, Missouri

James D. Pearson, MD
Assistant Professor of Anesthesiology
University of Alabama, Birmingham
University of Alabama Hospitals
Birmingham, Alabama

David R. Salter, MD, FRCSC
Assistant Professor of Surgery
Medical College of Virginia
Chief of Cardiothoracic Surgery
McGuire VA Medical Center
Richmond, Virginia

Lauraine M. Stewart, MD
Associate Professor
Department of Anesthesiology
Medical College of Virginia
Richmond, Virginia

Marc D. Thames, MD
Joseph T. Wearn University Professor
  in Medicine
Case Western Reserve University
  School of Medicine
Chief, Division of Cardiology
University Hospitals of Cleveland
Cleveland, Ohio

Contents

Preface

Ten years ago a monograph on organ transplantation would have been of interest to a minority of physicians at a few academic centers; today, however, organ transplantation is an accepted therapeutic modality. Heart and liver transplants are no longer newsworthy events, and lung transplants ultimately will become as commonplace.

Anesthesiologists who were already associated with organ transplant programs are being asked to meet greater challenges as our surgical colleagues find ways to perform transplants in patients who were previously considered inoperable. Because the number of transplant survivors is increasing exponentially, anesthesiologists who once thought organ transplantation did not concern their practices now are being asked to anesthetize post-transplant patients for unrelated surgical procedures. Finally, the economic impact of organ transplantation affects us all.

Although a monograph of this size certainly cannot provide exhaustive coverage of issues related to anesthesia and organ transplantation, we have attempted to provide a reasonable overview of anesthesiology for heart, lung, and liver transplantation. Because use of mechanical devices as a bridge to heart transplants is becoming more commonplace, an understanding of those devices is essential for the transplantation anesthesiologist. The physiology of the brain-dead donor, immunosuppressive therapy for the transplant recipient, and use of cardiopulmonary bypass in transplantation, although not directly related to anesthesia, nonetheless merit discussion because these conditions affect our patients and our management of them. Lastly, a frank discussion of the economic and ethical issues surrounding organ transplantation is an appropriate final chapter because this is an area that is all too often ignored, both locally and nationally.

I would like to thank Andrew Clark, Lauraine Stewart, and Richard

Wolman for carrying the extra clinical load imposed on them while I was working on this monograph. I also thank each of the authors for a job well done. Many of them consented to contribute to this effort in spite of an already heavy workload. Finally, I would like to give special thanks to Earl Wynands and Skip Ellison for their friendship, advice, and moral support.

Judith A. Fabian, MD

Joel J. Berberich

Anesthesia for Heart and Heart–Lung Transplantation

1 |

HEART TRANSPLANTATION

Cardiac transplantation has progressed from an experimental animal and clinical phase, conducted at a limited number of centers, to an accepted therapeutic modality with widespread practice. A technique for orthotopic transplantation of the heart was described by Lower and Shumway in dogs in 1960[1] and first performed in humans by Barnard in 1967.[2] Initial enthusiasm for the procedure was tempered when mortality rates approached 90%, primarily because of infection and rejection. Successes in the limited number of centers that continued to perform this procedure developed over the ensuing decade of the 1970s, primarily with the advent of improved immunosuppressive agents, especially cyclosporine. The next decade was marked by the growth and acceptance of heart transplantation as a valid clinical modality. A total of 117 heart transplants was performed throughout the United States in 1981. This number increased to 346 in 1984 and to 1688 in 1989. The 12-month survival rate for patients transplanted for the first time in 1988 was 82.8%. Currently, 151 centers in the United States are performing heart transplants.[3]

Reports of anesthetic experience in managing these patients have paralleled the development of the field surgically. Empiric observations in small numbers of patients were initially reported.[4–9] Subsequently, larger series of uncontrolled studies were reported.[10-15] More recently, limited controlled studies have been reported.[16] Anesthetic management of the heart transplant recipient has been reviewed recently, particularly in a definitive review by Clark and Martin.[17-19]

The Heart Donor

Heart transplant donors have suffered irreversible neurologic injury, usually from head trauma. Acute and chronic cardiac diseases that preclude donation must be eliminated by historical, physical, and clinical evaluations. A history of chest trauma, cardiac arrest, and hypotensive episodes should be absent, and use of inotropic support should be minimal. However, when echocardiography has additionally been employed for screening of donor hearts, some hearts that previously would have been rejected have been found to be satisfactory for transplantation.[20] Although younger donor hearts have been shown to afford better long-term recipient survival,[21] older donors are acceptable to enlarge the donor pool but usually require angiographic evidence of absence of coronary artery disease. Inspection of the donor heart on procurement remains the definitive assessment of acceptability for transplantation. Donor infectious processes, including viral ones, must be ruled out and recipient size and immunologic compatibility assured.

The brain-dead donor does not require anesthetic administration; however, muscle relaxants are commonly given. Nonetheless, anesthetic management of the brain-dead donor is not simple because of the need to maintain homeostasis in the face of failing homeostatic mechanisms and hemodynamic instability.[22] Adequate volume replacement is especially critical to donor management. Donor cardiectomy is coordinated with the harvesting of other organs. Optimal myocardial preservation techniques are still being investigated. Hypothermic preservation protocols, with and without cardioplegia, are the usual practice.[23-25] Most cardiac transplant centers prefer to limit the ischemic time of the donor heart to 4 hours or less (aortic cross-clamp placement in the recipient until aortic cross-clamp release in the donor). However, the true upper limit of this time is not known.[26] The British group at Harefield Hospital has sought to evaluate the donor heart more systematically. Darracott-Cankovic, using polarizing microscopy to evaluate the donor heart, has reported only a 6% recipient mortality with normal donor hearts vs. a 44% recipient mortality when structural abnormalities of the donor hearts were detected microscopically.[27]

The Heart Recipient

By definition, candidates for cardiac transplantation must be suffering from end-stage cardiac pump failure, unremedial to surgical modalities other than cardiac replacement.[28,29]

Recipient heart transplant selection criteria include the following:[19]

1. New York Heart Association class IV cardiac dysfunction unremedial to other therapy
2. One-year survival estimated to be less than 50%
3. Age less than 65 years
4. No systemic illness other than abnormalities related to heart failure
5. Emotional stability
6. Adequate psychosocial support system
7. Absence of:
   a. Pulmonary hypertension; pulmonary resistance less than 8 Woods units
   b. Severe, irreversible hepatic, renal, or pulmonary disease
   c. Active systemic or pulmonary infection
   d. Insulin-dependent diabetes mellitus (relative contraindication)
   e. History of uncontrollable hypertension
   f. Systemic vascular or cerebrovascular disease
   g. Active peptic ulcer disease
   h. Unresolved substance abuse

It is important to recognize that mortality without transplantation in this critically ill population is high, with 3-month mortality at Stanford exceeding 90%.[29,30]

The pathologic dysfunction of most cardiac transplant recipients is either primary congestive cardiomyopathy or ischemic cardiomyopathy secondary to coronary artery disease. These two diagnoses account for more than 90% of heart transplant recipients nationwide.[3] Patients with end-stage pump failure secondary to valvular pathology are usually excluded from the recipient pool because of their advanced age or their secondary pulmonary hypertension. Patients with restrictive cardiomyopathy due to infiltrative processes are usually excluded because of the subsequent disease involvement in the transplanted heart.[31] A limited number of adults, but an increasing pediatric population, receive heart transplants because of congenital heart disease. The specific problems in managing neonatal heart transplant patients have been reviewed recently by Martin and are presented in Chapter 2.[32] Only a limited number of adults receive cardiac transplantations for cardiac tumors or cardiac trauma.

Patients with insulin-dependent diabetes mellitus are relatively excluded from the recipient pool because of the difficulty with diabetic control in the face of steroid immunosuppression and probable exaggerated atherogenesis of the coronary vascular bed of the transplanted heart in these patients. One of the most limiting exclusion factors for recipients is the presence of pulmonary hypertension because of the acute load placed on the transplanted heart. Kormos has reported a mortality rate of 25% caused by right ventricular failure when the gradient between mean pulmonary artery and wedge pressure exceeds 15 mm Hg or the pulmonary vascular resistance exceeds 5 Woods units in recipients.[33]

The high relative risk for heart transplantation in patients with pulmonary hypertension has been confirmed and is widely accepted.[28,34] It should be noted that pulmonary hypertension may be reduced to acceptable levels for transplantation by conventional long-term therapy (diuretics, digitalis, and captopril) or acute pulmonary vasodilator therapy using various drug regimens. Isosorbide dinitrate has been found by one group to be more acceptable than either systemic nitroglycerin or sodium nitroprusside for reducing recipient pulmonary hypertension preoperatively.[35] Others have advocated the usefulness of amrinone as a selective pulmonary vasodilator.[36] Although once excluded on the basis of poor outcome, recipient age no longer appears to be an exclusionary factor for selection as a heart transplant recipient.[37]

Functionally, patients with either idiopathic or ischemic cardiomyopathy may be considered to be a subpopulation of a larger category: the dilated cardiomyopathies.[38,39] The hallmark of this disease process is ultimate deterioration in cardiac performance with inability to pump an adequate blood and oxygen supply to sustain organ function. Depression of pump performance is associated with activation of complex, interdependent, compensatory mechanisms that may initially be supportive in maintaining performance. In the long term, some of these effects may be deleterious and exacerbate decompensation.[40]

Myocardial contractility is impaired, causing depressed systolic performance, which is exacerbated by the altered geometry that results from ventricular dilatation.[41] Blood volume increases as a result of sodium and water retention from renin-angiotensin-aldosterone activation or decreased renal blood flow. Initially, the volume increase may improve pump function through the Frank-Starling mechanism. Ultimately, however, the preload reserve becomes exhausted, and no increase in stroke volume occurs with increased end diastolic volume in the dilated heart.[40]

Likewise, adrenergic activity initially increases with pump failure to augment contractility. However, chronic adrenergic activation leads to catecholamine depletion and decreased adrenergic receptors (down-regulation).[42] This process leads to depressed responsiveness to exogenous catecholamine agonists and to the higher circulating catecholamine levels usually present in these patients. Adrenergic activity may further depress renal blood flow and increase venous pressures, leading to increased pulmonary capillary hydrostatic pressure, which exacerbates pulmonary congestion. In addition, left ventricular impedance is increased, partly because of postsystolic elevation of wall stress.[43]

In response to the depression of stroke volume and decompensation of physiologic augmentation of stroke volume, patients with dilated cardiomyopathy develop a mild to moderate resting tachycardia.

Preoperative Assessment

Because of the time constraints associated with distant organ procurement and the coordination of donor and recipient matching, the anesthesiologist usually is aware of the impending transplant only a few hours before surgery, at best. As a result, preoperative evaluation is not aimed at therapeutic alterations, which hopefully have been optimized as much as possible by other specialists. Rather, assessment is aimed at evaluating the extent of cardiac and secondary organ dysfunction. Typically, two types of patients present for heart transplantation. One group is relatively compensated, though possibly requiring intravenous inotropic support. Patients in this group may even be ambulatory in a nonhospital environment.

The second group of patients is largely decompensated and possibly moribund. Typically, they may require mechanical ventilation or mechanical circulatory support. Mechanical circulatory support (e.g., intra-aortic balloon counter-pulsation, left or right ventricular assist devices, total artificial hearts) may be employed before heart transplantation. The primary indications for these are: inability to wean from cardiopulmonary bypass, acute cardiogenic shock secondary to myocardial infarction, and acute deterioration of a cardiomyopathic state.

The relative distribution of patients in the second group is subject to multiple institutional factors, with a 2% and 6% incidence in two series[12,44] vs. 13% and 22% in two other series.[30,45] In a survey of 34 institutions, Hensley has confirmed these institutional differences: 50% of institutions reported no patients who required mechanical assistance preoperatively; 38% reported 1% to 10% of patients who required assistance preoperatively; the remaining 12% of institutions reported 11% or more of patients who required mechanical circulatory assistance preoperatively.[14] It should be emphasized that the requirement for circulatory assistance in recipients appears to have no effect on the outcome of cardiac transplantation.[45,46]

Preoperative sedation is usually avoided secondary to its myocardial depression, especially since it may be synergistic with subsequent anesthetics.[14] In contrast, antacid therapy is commonly administered, since these patients may be at risk for acid aspiration due to delayed gastric emptying, recent food ingestion before the patient's notification of surgery, or administration of oral cyclosporine in a chocolate milk vehicle.

Monitoring

The usual intraoperative monitors are employed in cardiac transplantation. One area of controversy, however, is whether to monitor pulmonary artery pressure. In a 1986 survey, Hensley reported that 32% of reporting institutions employed pulmonary artery pressure monitoring in the prebypass period for cardiac transplantation and 44% in the postbypass period.[14] In this series, 15 of the 1273 patients failed to terminate bypass because of right ventricular failure and 12 because of biventricular failure, of a total of 33 patients failing to terminate bypass. Presumably, a pulmonary artery catheter may have assisted in the management of these 27 patients.

The arguments made against placing a pulmonary artery catheter are (1) the increased risk of infection in these immunocompromised patients; (2) the requirement for catheter withdrawal before recipient cardiectomy into a questionably sterile sleeve; and (3) the lack of any requirement for pulmonary artery pressure measurements in the absence of pulmonary hypertension.[4,7,12]

Recently, some investigators have suggested that, rather than the usual pulmonary artery catheter, a modified right ventricular ejection fraction catheter should be employed. This special catheter is equipped with a fast-response thermistor (50 milliseconds) that measures beat-to-beat variation in pulmonary artery blood temperature and allows calculation of right ventricular ejection.[47,48] Right ventricular monitoring helped demonstrate the continuing need for postoperative pharmacologic support of the right ventricle in patients who had normal pulmonary vascular resistance before their transplantation.

Especially with the advent of cyclosporine as the mainstay of immunosuppression, endomyocardial biopsy has become the standard for evaluating postoperative organ rejection.[49] Since the patient's right internal jugular vein is usually employed for repeated access for this procedure, some groups prefer to employ the left internal jugular vein for intraoperative central venous access. Sterility in the placement of this and all vascular catheters in transplant patients should be meticulously maintained. Although some institutions prefer to employ sterile laryngoscope equipment and anesthesia circuits, no data support the benefit of these added steps.

Limited data exist concerning the risk or benefits of intraoperative transesophageal echocardiographic monitoring for cardiac transplantation.[50] However, a limited series supported its special utility for monitoring right ventricular function on a continuing basis after transplantation.[51]

Anesthetic Management

Anesthetic induction must balance the competing risks of further myocardial depression from relative or absolute anesthetic drug overdoses vs. the risk of aspiration pneumonitis in patients with full stomachs. Anesthetic management is not uniquely different from that of managing the patient with end-stage cardiomyopathy for other cardiac and noncardiac operations.

The anesthetist conducting the first heart transplant reported that, "It was not anticipated that we would be faced with anything that we had not been faced with before, and the anesthesia was conducted with optimism. In fact, things went very much as expected and we were not compelled to do anything of a startling nature."[8] This statement illustrates the point that cardiovascular anesthesiologists are experienced in managing patients with ventricular dysfunction. The differences in managing the heart transplant recipient are limited.

One major difference in managing these cardiomyopathic patients for heart transplantation does exist. Since the recipient's own heart will no longer be employed after the transplant, one may afford to use drugs to augment its function before cardiopulmonary bypass to optimize other nonregenerative organ functions (e.g., brain, kidney) and to control pulmonary hypertension. Potential adverse effects on the heart, which would limit management in other circumstances, are not a concern since the heart will be removed.

Many different intravenous agents have been used for induction of anesthesia. For the first heart transplantations and early series of heart transplantations, thiopental sodium was the most commonly used agent.[5,7,8] More recently, anesthesiologists have employed different induction agents; some have used a classic rapid sequence induction with either ketamine or etomidate (18% of surveyed institutions).[14] However, the down-regulation of adrenergic receptors may theoretically unmask the negative inotropic properties of ketamine. In one randomized series of heart transplant patients, ketamine (1.5 mg/kg) resulted in a 28% increase in mean arterial pressure, but with a 109% increase in central venous pressure and an 84% increase in pulmonary capillary wedge pressure.[16] Cardiac index was unaffected in this series, but these results indicate that less myocardial work occurred at the expense of higher wall tension. Although there were no outcome differences, and clinical experience is not reported to be adverse, evidence from this study warrants cautious use of ketamine for heart transplantation. In a series of patients with advanced congestive heart failure who were not undergoing heart transplantation, etomidate, but not midazolam, was found to be acceptable for inducing anesthesia.[52]

Other anesthesiologists have elected to induce anesthesia with high-dose opioids with or without benzodiazepines. This technique was employed by two thirds of the institutions surveyed in 1986.[14] Both classic rapid-sequence induction and a modified rapid-sequence induction with cricoid pressure have been employed. Drug dosage is decreased because of delayed drug effect from the prolonged circulation time, the smaller volume of distribution, and the depressed pharmacodynamic response.

In general, most heart transplant recipients tolerate anesthetic induction well. It has been suggested that when ventricular dysfunction occurs, it is primarily a consequence of increased systemic or pulmonary vascular resistance.[44] This occurrence is often reflected as an increase in central venous pressure. Coronary artery perfusion may decrease in response to the decrease in stroke volume of these patients.[53]

Although inhaled agents are less commonly employed, presumably due to their direct myocardial depression,[14] no outcome differences were noted in a retrospective review that compared inhaled anesthetics to opioids.[12] Inhaled agents were associated with a greater frequency of hypotension, but dysrhythmia occurred more frequently in heart transplant patients who received opioids as the maintenance anesthetic. In one retrospective series, no obvious reason was found to recommend fentanyl citrate over sufentanil as the opioid of choice for anesthetic maintenance for heart transplantation.[11] Delayed narcotic clearance, due to intrinsic hepatic dysfunction and hepatic hypoperfusion, theoretically could increase the incidence of prolonged postoperative mechanical ventilation with its attendant risk of infection. However, this possibility does not appear to be a problem.[11,12,14] Although nitrous oxide has been used for heart transplant patients,[7] it is usually avoided because of its potential to produce myocardial depression and pulmonary hypertension.

In summary, the choice of agent appears less important than the ability to control hemodynamics in this patient population with limited reserve. Hemodynamic support may need to be increased or alternate therapy employed to avoid further cardiac decompensation in the pre-bypass period. In addition, volume and blood product support may be required in the prebypass period because of the increasing frequency with which cardiac transplant patients have had previous median sternotomies.

The management of cardiopulmonary bypass in these patients is not different, except that rewarming is usually prolonged because of the more profound cooling of the donor heart and the ischemia time, which is more prolonged than the usual cardiac operation.

The transplanted heart is controlled by the donor sinoatrial node, which is excluded from all normal autonomic innervation. Although a second recipient P wave may be seen on the electrocardiogram, this is nonfunctional. Typically, the transplanted heart develops a sinus bradycardia or atrioventricular block. Thus, chronotropic support is essential for patient management. Oxygen delivery strongly depends on heart rate in these patients because of a fixed stroke volume. Ventricular pacing may be an acceptable modality but affords no hemodynamic support other than heart rate control. In contrast, isoproterenol or dobutamine are more commonly employed for postoperative support because of their additional potential to augment contractility and to decrease pulmonary hypertension. Indeed, myocardial contractility often is depressed initially in the newly transplanted heart.[54]

Echocardiography has demonstrated decreased right ventricular dimensions, increased left ventricular posterior wall thickness (myocardial edema), and biatrial enlargement.[55] The decrease in diastolic compliance necessitates elevated ventricular filling pressures. It is essential to maintain this volume load since the denervated heart is isolated from the baroreceptor control loop and is unable to increase heart rate or cardiac output in response to hypovolemia. No special problems have been reported in the transfusion of autologous blood after cardiopulmonary bypass in heart transplant patients to augment their intravascular volume.[56] Intrinsic blood volume regulation may be altered in these patients, further necessitating adequate volume loading.[57]

Even in the apparent absence of pulmonary hypertension in the transplant recipient preoperatively, right ventricular dysfunction commonly develops after cardiopulmonary bypass.[50,55,58,60] This is usually self-limiting over a period of days. Clinical management of right ventricular failure is not different in these patients. Specific management with prostaglandin as a pulmonary vasodilator has been effective.[59,60] Amrinone may also have some selective use in managing this problem.

TABLE 1-1. Comparison of Effects of Direct- and Indirect-Acting Drugs on Heart Rate and Blood Pressure in Patients With Normal and Denervated Hearts

Drug	Action	Heart Rate		Blood Pressure	
		N	D	N	D
Anticholinergics	I	↑	—	—	—
Anticholinesterases	I	↓	—	—	—
Propranolol	D	↓	↓	—	—
Verapamil	D	↓	↓	↓	↓
Ephedrine	D & I	↑	± ↑	↑	± ↑
Pancuronium	I	↑	—	—	—
Phenylephrine	D	↓	—	↑	↑

I, indirect; D, direct; N, normal; D, denervated. (Adapted from Baum V: Anesthesia for heart and heart-lung transplantation. In Kapoor AS, Laks H, Schroeder J, Yacoub M (eds): Cardiomyopathies and Cardiopulmonary Transplantation. New York, McGraw Hill, 1990)

The consequences of cardiac denervation are reviewed elsewhere in this monograph (see Chapter 3). A few points that affect postbypass management should be included here (Table 1-1).[61] Response to direct β-adrenergic agonists is qualitatively unchanged.[62] In fact, sensitivity to isoproterenol may be increased because of receptor up-regulation.[63] In contrast, cardiac responses to drugs that indirectly release catecholamines (e.g., tyramine, dopamine, ephedrine, metaraminol, mephentermine) are diminished but not abolished. However, clinical differences with the use of dopamine and ephedrine in these patients appear to be minimal. Likewise, drugs with anticholinergic effects (e.g., atropine, pancuronium bromide) have no effect on heart rate or atrioventricular conduction.

HEART–LUNG TRANSPLANTATION

Combined heart–lung transplantation has been used as a therapeutic modality for patients with end-stage pulmonary vascular disease. The first human heart–lung transplant was performed in 1968 by Cooley.[64] Even more than isolated cardiac transplantation, there was a hiatus in performance of this operation until the advent of improved immunosuppression.[65] Shumway led the resurgence of this procedure in 1981 and has documented continuing improved results.[66]

Anesthetic management for combined heart–lung transplantation has been reviewed recently.[67,68] In 1989, 67 heart–lung transplants were performed in the United States. The 12-month survival for patients transplanted for the first time was 56.9% in 1989. Currently, 81 centers are listed as performing heart–lung transplants in the United States.[3]

The Heart–Lung Donor

In addition to meeting acceptable criteria for cardiac transplantation, heart–lung donors also must have satisfactory pulmonary function. In particular, since most donors are trauma victims, chest trauma and pulmonary contusions should not be present. Likewise, aspiration pneumonitis and neurogenic pulmonary edema should be absent. In general, satisfactory gas exchange at an inspired oxygen concentration of less than 40% with normal pulmonary compliance is required. Only 20% of potential cardiac donors also have acceptable lungs for transplantation.[67] In addition, donor and recipient size compatibility is more difficult, since not only gross body weights but also thoracic cavity sizes and dimensions must be comparable.

Donor anesthetic management is similar, except for the use of a pulmonary vasodilator and lung preservation perfusate.[69] Distant organ procurement has become more commonplace. Previously, the availability of organs was limited when only local procurement was available because of problems with consent for transportation of the donor. Nonetheless, locally procured organs may be preferable, since more frequent support with pulmonary vasodilators and diuretics and poorer respiratory gas exchange have been reported with distantly procured organs.[70]

The Heart–Lung Recipient

Candidates for heart–lung transplantation have end-stage parenchymal lung or pulmonary vascular disease that is unresponsive to medical therapy and not treatable by other surgical approaches. Pulmonary hypertension usually precludes treatment with an isolated cardiac transplant; likewise, unilateral lung transplant may not be a viable option with poor right ventricular function.

The vast majority of recipients suffer from pulmonary vascular disease, usually primary pulmonary hypertension or Eisenmenger's syndrome. A minority of patients have obstructive, restrictive, or destructive lung parenchymal disease, with cystic fibrosis patients being the most common in this group. Patients with pulmonary hypertension secondary to chronic recurrent pulmonary emboli cannot be successfully treated with heart–lung transplantation.

Patients with pulmonary vascular disease develop a resting hypoxemia that is often compensated, but with marked exertional dyspnea. In addition to ventilation and perfusion abnormalities, interpulmonary right-to-left shunting may exacerbate the hypoxemia in the few heart–lung transplantation patients with chronic obstructive lung disease. Most recipients have a restrictive ventilatory pattern associated with their primary pulmonary hypertension or from their primary pulmonary disease. These patients have a decreased pulmonary compliance, increased residual volume, and abnormal small airway flow.[67]

Pulmonary hypertension with near-systemic pressures is common in these patients, with a low cardiac output state on the basis of either right or biventricular failure. Patients usually receive supplemental oxygen preoperatively but are not commonly mechanically ventilated. Diuretics are employed, but metabolic alkalosis is carefully avoided to prevent further exacerbation of pulmonary hypertension. Although digoxin is commonly given, some feel it is contraindicated because of a potential exacerbation of pulmonary hypertension.[71] Rather, various vasodilator therapies have been employed to control the pulmonary hypertension preoperatively. Multiple drug regimens may be used because of the marked differences in individual responsiveness to pulmonary vasodilators in this patient population.[72,73] Most recently, prostacyclin infusions have been employed as an aggressive, but costly, short-term modality to attempt to stabilize pulmonary hemodynamics in these patients before the heart–lung transplantation.[74] The patients may also be systemically anticoagulated with Coumadin,[75] but, if not, frequently receive low-dose heparin therapy or antiplatelet drugs.

Anesthetic monitoring is much the same as for heart transplantation, but the benefits of pulmonary artery catheterization may be more apparent. However, some experienced groups believe that, since pulmonary artery pressures usually decline to normal levels in the transplanted heart and lung, central venous pressure monitoring is adequate in the postbypass phase.

Potential problems with anesthetic induction are at least as severe as for the heart transplant recipient. Although patients have a full stomach, a true rapid-sequence induction may exacerbate the underlying high pulmonary vascular resistance, further depressing cardiac output and resulting in decompensation. Thus, in spite of a potential full stomach, a controlled, modified rapid-sequence induction may be more advisable. Anesthetic induction techniques are similar to those employed in the heart-transplant patient, with the exception that ketamine is contra-indicated because of its elevation of pulmonary vascular resistance.[76]

After induction, the endotracheal tube is inserted with the cuff placed just beyond the vocal cords. Cuff occlusion pressure should be monitored to avoid potential ischemia of this poorly vascularized area near the planned tracheal anastomosis.

Anesthesia is usually maintained with high-dose opioids because of the potentially deleterious effects of systemic vasodilation from inhaled agents. Nitrous oxide is avoided because of potential hypoxemia from the reduction in the fraction of inspired oxygen and because of its potential to increase pulmonary vascular resistance.[77] Ventilation should be adjusted to avoid exacerbation of pulmonary vascular resistance by either hypoxemia or hypercarbia.

Manipulation of vasodilator therapy to optimize pulmonary vascular dynamics is extremely risky in these patients because of the lability and unpredictability of the responses. Intensive treatment may result in systemic vasodilation, which may in turn lead to refractory bradycardia with a depression in cardiac output unresponsive to fluids or drugs. Attempts at treatment with systemic vasoconstrictors may actually worsen matters by increasing pulmonary vasoconstriction. Systemic vasodilation, on the other hand, may precipitate a transient reflex increase in cardiac output, exacerbating pulmonary hypertension and increasing right ventricular work, leading to cardiac failure. In addition, systemic hypotension may also decrease coronary artery perfusion pressures and the resultant ischemia may further exacerbate right ventricular failure.[72] Sinoatrial and atrioventricular node ischemia may give rise to poorly tolerated cardiac rhythm disturbances. It is clear that avoidance of decreased systemic vascular resistance is essential to the management of these patients.

The cardiopulmonary bypass period is similar to other cardiac operations. A few specific points should be mentioned. Repositioning of the endotracheal tube may be required for the tracheal anastomosis. In addition, absence of a leak at this anastomosis must be verified. Frequent, but cautious, pulmonary toilet is employed after completion of the tracheal anastomosis to suction blood clots and other secretions. Ventilation is initiated toward the end of the bypass phase, but the fraction of inspired oxygen is kept at 50% or as low as possible to maintain adequate oxygenation; this percentage is used because of the accepted, but not well documented, risk of oxygen toxicity in the transplanted lung.[67] Prophylactic positive end-expiratory pressure of 0.5 to 1 kPa is commonly used to decrease pulmonary atelectasis.

Weaning from bypass is analogous to that for cardiac transplantation, with the same need to support the recently denervated heart with fluid and chronotropic therapies. Maintenance of adequate intravascular volume and filling pressures is often more difficult because of the increased bleeding associated with this procedure. Extensive collateral and bronchial circulation often has developed in these patients. A particular emphasis is made by the surgeon to assure adequate posterior mediastinal hemostasis in the initial phases of dissection and organ attachment, since this area is virtually inaccessible after the suturing of the donor heart and lungs. Blood products are typically required in the postbypass period to maintain intravascular volume and as procoagulants.

In contrast to the effects of denervation on the heart, the effects of denervation of the lung on anesthetic management immediately after the transplant are limited, if any. Ventilatory function of the transplanted lungs resumes postoperatively, and the patient may be extubated after recovery from the anesthetic. Bilateral vagotomy in awake humans does not affect resting tidal volume and rate, but end-tidal carbon dioxide at the end of maximal breath holding is elevated.[78] Ventilatory response to hypocarbia may be depressed in some of these patients.[67,79]

Most important, the cough reflex is not elicited by stimuli distal to the anastomosis.[78,80] Patients must, therefore, be awake enough to respond to verbal commands to cough, especially patients at increased risk for aspiration because of left recurrent laryngeal nerve dysfunction from mechanical effects of the enlarged pretransplant pulmonary artery. Vagotomy produces bronchodilation and inhibits the bronchoconstrictive response to distal airway stimuli.[78,80] Despite this fact, bronchospasm can develop in these patients, presumably because of pharmacologic mechanisms independent of neural control. In at least one case, this bronchospasm was refractory to management in the immediate postbypass period.[81] Later, bronchospasm may be a manifestation of rejection of the transplanted lung.

In addition to severing nerve supply to the lungs, lymphatic drainage is also severed during heart–lung transplantation. Prevention of accumulation of lung water is managed by aggressive use of diuretics and limitation of crystalloid infusion throughout the perioperative period. The phenomenon of interstitial fluid accumulation is termed *reimplantation pulmonary edema.* This process affects pulmonary gas exchange in most patients.[82] The amount of urine production with forced diuresis has been shown to correlate well with alveolar-arterial oxygen tension gradients in heart–lung transplant recipients postoperatively.[70] In some patients, the reimplantation pulmonary edema response may also represent pulmonary rejection, which requires treatment with immunosuppression.

CONCLUSION

What was once a rare procedure confined to a few medical centers has become commonplace. Anesthesiologists who never expected to be challenged with heart and heart–lung transplant recipients are called on to exercise their skills not only for the actual transplantation, but for unrelated surgical procedures in patients who have had transplants. Sound knowledge of the physiology involved and thorough preparation will enable the anesthesiologist to help provide a safe intraoperative course.

References

1. Lower RR, Shumway NE: Studies on orthotopic transplantation of the canine heart. Surgical Forum 11:18, 1960
2. Barnard CW: A human cardiac transplant: An interim report of a successful operation performed at Groote-Schur Hospital, Capetown. S Afr Med J 41:1271, 1967
3. United Network for Organ Sharing: Transplant Statistics 1991
4. Farman JK: Anesthesia for cardiac transplantation. Cleve Clin Q 48:142, 1981
5. Fernando NA, Keenan RL, Boyan CP: Anesthetic experience with cardiac transplantation. J Thorac Cardiovasc Surg 75:531, 1978
6. Harrison JA, Bailey RG, Thomsen PG: A heart transplantation. IV. Anesthetic and cardiopulmonary bypass. Med J Aust 1:670, 1969
7. Keats AS, Strong MJ, Girgis KZ et al: Observations during anesthesia for cardiac homotransplantation in ten patients. Anesthesiology 30:192, 1969
8. Ozinsky J: Cardiac transplantation: The anaesthetist's view: A case report. S Afr Med J 41:1268, 1967
9. Wielhorski WA, Paiement V, Dyrda I, Grondin P: The performance of nine human hearts before, during and after transplantation. Can Anaesth Soc J 17:97, 1970
10. Alvaraz J, Casas I, Litvan H, Villar-Landeira JM: Manejo anestesico en el trasplante cardiaco. Rev Esp Cardiol 40:31, 1987
11. Berberich JJ, Fabian JA: A retrospective analysis of fentanyl and sufentanil for cardiac transplantation. J Cardiothoracic Anesthesia 1:200, 1987
12. Demas K, Wyner J, Mihm FG et al: Anaesthesia for heart transplantation: A retrospective study and review. Br J Anaesth 58:1357, 1986
13. Grebenik CR, Robinson PN: Cardiac transplantation at Harefield. Anaesthesia 40:131, 1985
14. Hensley FA Jr, Martin DE, Larach DR, Romanoff ME: Anesthetic management for cardiac transplantation in North America—1986 survey. J Cardiothoracic Anesthesia 1:429, 1987
15. Schaps VD, Alken A, Mahler D: Anasthesiologische erfahrungen bei 199 herztransplantationen. Anaesthesiol Reanim 14:89, 1989
16. Gutzke GE, Shah KB, Glisson SN et al: Cardiac transplantation: A prospective comparison of ketamine and sufentanil for anesthetic induction. J Cardiothoracic Anesthesia 3:389, 1989

17. Baum VC: Anesthesia for heart transplantation recipient. Seminars in Anesthesia 4:298, 1990
18. Clark NJ, Martin RD: Anesthetic considerations for patients undergoing cardiac transplantation. J Cardiothoracic Anesthesia 2:519, 1988
19. Gallo JA Jr, Cork RC: Anesthesia for cardiac transplantation. Contemp Anesth Pract 10:91, 1987
20. Gilbert EM, Krueger JK, Murray JN et al: Echocardiographic evaluation of potential cardiac transplant donors. J Thorac Cardiovasc Surg 95:1003, 1988
21. Gao SZ, Schroeder J, Alderman E et al: Clinical and laboratory correlates of accelerated coronary vascular disease in the cardiac transplant patient. Circulation (suppl II):219A, 1986
22. Wetzel RC, Setzer N, Stiff JL et al: Hemodynamic responses in brain dead organ donor patients. Anesth Analg 64:125, 1985
23. Keon WJ, Hendry PJ, Taichman GC: Cardiac transplantation: The ideal myocardial temperature for graft transport. Ann Thorac Surg 46:337, 1988
24. Mollhof T, Sukehiro S, Flameng W, VanAken H: Preservation of donor hearts: Influence of cardioplegic solution on myocardial high energy phosphate content (abstr). Anesthesiology 21:A630, 1989
25. Mollhof T, Sukehiro S, Flameng W, VanAken H: Successful transplantation of dog hearts after 24 hours of cold storage (abstr). Anesthesiology 73:A628, 1990
26. Copeland JG, Jones M, Spragg R et al: In-vitro preservation of canine hearts for 24 to 48 hours followed by successful orthotopic transplantation. Ann Surg 178:687, 1973
27. Darracott-Cankovic S, Stovin PG, Wheeldon D et al: Effect of donor heart damage on survival after transplantation. Eur J Cardiothorac Surg 3:525, 1989
28. Copeland JG, Emery RW, Levinson MM et al: Selection of patients for cardiac transplantation. Circulation 75:2, 1987
29. Evans RW, Maier AM: Outcome of patients referred for cardiac transplantation. J Am Coll Cardiol 8:1312, 1986
30. Pennock JL, Oyer PE, Reitz BA et al: Cardiac transplantation in perspective for the future. J Thorac Cardiovasc Surg 83:168, 1982
31. Conner R, Hosenpud J, Norman D et al: Recurrence of amyloidosis in a cardiac allograft. J Heart Transplant 5:385, 1986
32. Martin RD, Parisi F, Robinson TW, Bailey L: Anesthetic management of neonatal cardiac transplantation. J Cardiothoracic Anesthesia 3:465, 1989
33. Kormos RL, Thompson M, Hardesty RL et al: Utility of preoperative right heart catheterization data as a predictor of survival after heart transplantation. J Heart Transplant 5:391, 1986
34. Kirklin JK, Naften OC, McGiffin DC et al: Analysis of morbid events and risk factors for death after cardiac transplantation. J Am Coll Cardiol 11:917, 1988
35. Curling PE, Dobbs SG, Psyhojus TJ, Kanter KR, Lattouf OM, Baumann DI: Evaluation of patients with pulmonary hypertension for orthotopic heart transplantation: Nitroprusside vs. isosorbide dinitrate (abstr). Anesth Analg 68:S67, 1989
36. Deeb GM, Bolling SF: The role of amrinone in potential heart transplantation with pulmonary hypertension. J Cardiothoracic Anesthesia 3:33, 1989

37. Carrier M, Emory RW, Riley JE et al: Cardiac transplantation in patients over 50 years of age. J Am Coll Card 8:285, 1986
38. Johnson RA, Palacios I: Dilated cardiomyopathies of the adult. N Engl J Med 307:1051, 1982
39. O'Connell JB, Gunnar RM: Dilated congested cardiomyopathy: Prognostic features and therapy. J Heart Transplant 2:7, 1982
40. Parmley WW: Pathophysiology of congestive heart failure. Am J Cardiol 56:7A, 1985
41. Grossman W, Braunwald E, Mann T: Contractile state of the left ventricle in man as evaluated from end systolic pressure-volume relationships. Circulation 56:845, 1977
42. Bristow MR, Ginsburg R, Miobe W et al: Decreased catecholamine sensitivity and beta adrenergic receptor density in failing human hearts. N Engl J Med 307:205, 1982
43. Weber KT, Janicki JS: The heart as a muscle pump system and the concept of heart failure. Am Heart J 98:371, 1979
44. Dikel ND, Gruber TJ, Watkins JE, Estrin JA: Determinants of ventricular performance during induction of anesthesia of heart transplant recipients (abstr). Anesthesiology 73:A107, 1990
45. O'Connell JB, Renlund DJ, Robinson JA et al: Effect of preoperative hemodynamic support on survival following cardiac transplantation. Circulation (suppl III):78, 1988
46. Bolman RM III, Spray TL, Cox Jl et al: Heart transplantation in patients requiring preoperative mechanical support. J Heart Transplant 6:273, 1987
47. Gasior T, Armitage J, Stein K, Jacquet L, Miyamoto Y: Right ventricular performance in the transplanted heart (abstr). Anesthesiology 71:A86, 1989
48. Nakatsuka M, Colquhoun AD, Barnhart G: Right ventricular function of the denervated heart immediately after heart transplantation (abstr). Presented at the Society of Cardiovascular Anesthesia, Orlando, FL 1989
49. Caves PK, Billingham ME, Stinson ED, Shumway NE: Serial transvenous endomyocardial biopsy of the transplanted human heart: Improved management of acute rejection episodes. Lancet 1:821, 1974
50. Bhatia SJ, Kirshenbaum JM, Shemin RJ et al: Time course of resolution of pulmonary hypertension and right ventricular remodeling after orthotopic cardiac transplantation. Circulation 76:819, 1987
51. Curling PE, Michelson LG, Kanter Kr, Lattouf OM, Weintraub WS, Waller JL: Monitoring orthotopic heart transplantation with 2-D transesophageal echocardiography and color flow mapping (abstr). Presented at the Society of Cardiovascular Anesthesia, Orlando, FL 1989
52. MacGillivray RG, Rocke DA, Mahomedy AE: Midazolam for induction of anaesthesia in patients with limited cardiac reserve: A comparison with etomidate. S Afr Med J 73:101, 1988
53. Estrin JA, Gruber Tj, Lora D, Watkins JE: Significance of the fall in coronary artery perfusion pressure during induction of anesthesia in heart transplant recipients (abstr). Presented at the Society of Cardiovascular Anesthesia, Orlando, FL 1989
54. Stinson EB, Caves PK, Griepp RB et al: Hemodynamic observations in the period after human heart transplantation. J Thorac Cardiovasc Surg 69:264, 1975
55. Hosenpud JD, Norman DJ, Cobanoglu A et al: Serial echocardiographic

findings early after heart transplantation: Evidence for reversible right ventricular dysfunction and myocardial edema. J Heart Transplant 6:343, 1987

56. Sorbara C, Dan M, Dona B, Bonato R, Gallucci V, Giron GP: Autotransfusion of intraoperative blood losses during cardiopulmonary bypass in orthotopic heart transplantation (abstr). Presented at the Society of Cardiovascular Anesthesia, Orlando, FL 1989

57. Hertz SN, Fusezi L, Iberti TJ, Smith CR: Atrial natriuretic factor secretion in cardiac transplantation (abstr). Anesthesiology 71:A190, 1989

58. Gierarts R, Schertz C, Ghignone M: Right ventricular failure after heart transplantation caused by a kink in the pulmonary artery anastomosis. J Cardiothorac Anesth 4:470, 1989

59. Fonger JD, Borkon AM, Baumgartner WA et al: Acute right ventricular failure following heart transplantation: Improvement with prostaglandin E_1 and right ventricular assist. J Heart Transplant 5:317, 1986

60. Weiss CI, Bolman RM: Hemodynamic effects of prostaglandin E_1 in pulmonary hypertensive patients undergoing cardiac transplantation (abstr). Presented at the Society of Cardiovascular Anesthesia, Orlando, FL 1989

61. Baum V: Anesthesia for heart and heart–lung transplantation. In Kapoor AS, Laks H, Schroeder J, Yacoub M (eds): Cardiomyopathies and Cardiopulmonary Transplantation, p. New York, McGraw Hill, 1990

62. Cannom DS, Rider AK, Stinson EB et al: Electrophysiologic studies in the denervated human heart. II. Response to norepinephrine, isoproterenol and propanolol. Am J Cardiol 36:859, 1975

63. Yosuf S, Theodoropoulos S, Mathas CJ et al: Increased sensitivity of the denervated transplanted human heart to isoprenaline both before and after beta adrenergic blockage. Circulation 75:696, 1987

64. Cooley DA, Bloodwell RD, Halman GI, Nora JJ, Harrison GM, Leachman RD: Organ transplantation for advanced cardiopulmonary disease. Ann Thorac Surg 8:30, 1969

65. Reitz BA, Wallwork JL, Hunt SL et al: Heart/lung transplantation: Successful therapy for patients with pulmonary vascular disease. N Engl J Med 306:557, 1982

66. McCarthy PM, Starnes VA, Theodore J, Stinson EB, Oyer BE, Shumway NE: Improved survival following heart lung transplantation. J Thorac Cardiovasc Surg 99:54, 1990

67. Finch EJ, Jamieson SW: Anesthesia for combined heart and lung transplantation. Contemp Anesth Pract 10:109, 1987

68. Sale JP, Patel D, Duncan B, Waters JH: Anaesthesia for combined heart and lung transplantation. Anaesthesia 42:249, 1987

69. Ladowski JS, Hardesty RL, Griffith BP: Protection of the heart-lung allograft during procurement. J Heart Transplant 3:351, 1984

70. Norgaard M, McGlinch BP, Dikel ND, Estrin JA: Effects of fluid balance and prostaglandin E_1 (PGE1) on reimplantation pulmonary edema in heart-lung transplant recipients (abstr). Anesthesiology 73:A1189, 1990

71. Coates AL, Desmond K, Asher MI, Hortop J, Beaudry PH: The effect of digoxin on exercise capacity and exercising cardiac function in cystic fibrosis. Chest 82:54B, 1982

72. Palevsky HI, Fisman AP: The management of primary pulmonary hypertension. JAMA 265:1014, 1991

73. Hermiller JB, Bambach D, Thompson MJ et al: Vasodilators and prostaglandin inhibitors in primary pulmonary hypotension. Ann Intern Med 97:480, 1982
74. Rubin LJ, Mendoza J, Hood M et al: Treatment of primary pulmonary hypertension with continuous intravenous prostacyclin (Epoprostenol). Ann Intern Med 112:485, 1990
75. Furter V, Steele PM, Edwards WD, Gersh BJ, McGoun MD, Frye RL: Primary pulmonary hypotension: Natural history and the importance of thrombosis. Circulation 70:580, 1984
76. White PF, Way WL, Trevor AJ: Ketamine: Its pharmacology and therapeutic uses. Anesthesiology 65:119, 1982
77. Schulte-Sasse Y, Hess W, Tarnow J: Pulmonary vascular response to nitrous oxide in patients with normal and high pulmonary vascular resistance. Anesthesiology 57:9, 1982
78. Nadel JA: Adoration of the vagi? N Engl J Med 311:463, 1984
79. Guz A, Nobel MIM, Widdicombe JG et al: The role of vagal and glossopharyngeal afferent nerves in respiratory sensation, control of breathing and arterial pressure regulation. Clin Sci 30:161, 1966
80. Richardson JB: Nerve supply to the lungs. Am Rev Respir Dis 119:785, 1979
81. Casella ES, Humphrey LS: Bronchospasm after cardiopulmonary bypass in a heart-lung transplant recipient. Anesthesiology 69:135, 1988
82. Theodre J, Jamiesson SW, Burke CM et al: Physiologic aspects of human heart-lung transplantation: Pulmonary function status of the post transplanted lung. Chest 86:349, 1984

Robert D. Martin
Martin W. Allard
The Loma Linda University Pediatric Heart
   Transplant Group

2 | Pediatric Cardiac Transplantation

Major advances in human cardiac transplantation have brought about its transition from an experimental procedure to an effective therapeutic modality.[1-3] Orthotopic cardiac transplantation provides definitive treatment for end-stage heart disease; in properly selected candidates, it not only relieves symptoms and improves functional status, but it also prolongs life expectancy.[4-8] This latter result is difficult to achieve with medical therapy alone.[9] Consequently, orthotopic cardiac transplantation has become an increasingly attractive therapeutic alternative for appropriate candidates with terminal cardiac disease and intractable heart failure. This remarkable achievement brings to fruition decades of basic and clinical research.

Cardiac transplantation is being performed in children and teenagers as a means to treat end-stage cardiac disease that it not responsive to medical treatment and for which no other surgical treatment is available.[10-14] Before cardiopulmonary bypass was available, only palliative operations could be performed on children with congenital heart defects. With cardiopulmonary bypass came the ability to replace components of the heart in children. Septal defects could be easily repaired, and valves and major arteries could be replaced.

The next logical progression was transplantation of the heart. In 1967 Kantrowitz performed an orthotopic transplant on a 1-month old infant.[15] Cooley performed the first cardiopulmonary transplantation on a 2-month old infant in 1968.[16] Because effective immunosuppressive agents were not then available, the survival rates in these early series were poor, and most centers discontinued their transplant programs.

Since the development of powerful immunosuppressive agents such as cyclosporine, the number of patients to undergo heart transplantation has steadily increased, and the indications for heart transplantation have been enlarged. Loma Linda University Medical Center has performed more than 100 cardiac transplantations on children younger than 1 year of age with survival in excess of 80% at 1 year or longer.

In 1984, when Bailey transplanted a baboon heart into a newborn infant who survived 20 days, the feasibility of neonatal heart transplantation was evident.[17] An important derivative of the xenotransplantation project has been the markedly increased awareness of the potential benefits of organ transplantation during neonatal life and the need for newborn human organs. With increasing numbers of pediatric heart transplants being performed worldwide, the evidence suggests that this procedure can be successful and that good quality of life can be achieved.

RECIPIENT INCLUSION CRITERIA

The protocol at Loma Linda University Medical Center requires that infants must have a gestation age greater than 36 weeks and birth weight greater than 2200 g. These criteria are to ensure adequate size of the right and left pulmonary arteries. Neonates unresponsive to prostaglandin (PGE_1) may require systemic-to-pulmonary shunts while awaiting a donor. The recipient must undergo a cardiac evaluation to confirm a diagnosis of hypoplastic left heart syndrome or other complex congenital heart disease for which no standardized treatment exists.[18]

Cardiac malformations that may be amenable to therapy by heart transplantation include the following:

1. Hypoplastic left heart syndrome (hypoplastic aortic tract complex)
2. Symptomatic severe Ebstein's anomaly with normal pulmonary arteries
3. Multiple obstructive rhabdomyoma
4. Pulmonary atresia/intact ventricular septum (large sinusoids)
5. Hypoplastic left heart equivalent: D-transposition with hypoplastic right ventricle and aortic tract; single ventricle with hypoplastic aortic tract; L-transposition with single ventricle and heart block
6. Severe congenital or acquired cardiomyopathy
7. Atrioventricular canal with hypoplastic left ventricle and mitral component (frequently associated with coarctation)

8. Single ventricle with subaortic obstruction (bulboventricular foramen)
9. Severe intrauterine atrioventricular valve insufficiency and ventricular dysfunction (see #2 for L-transposition)
10. Straddling atrioventricular valve and tensor apparatus
11. Complex truncus arteriosus

The diagnosis of end-stage cardiomyopathy must be made by the attending pediatrician or pediatric cardiologist. Echocardiography or heart catheterization confirmation is also helpful.

The recipient must be in stable metabolic and hemodynamic status while receiving PGE$_1$ and other supportive measures such as cardiac inotropic drugs, mechanical ventilation, parenteral nutrition, and so forth. All recipients receive a psychosocial evaluation. It is required that the candidate reside within 45 minutes traveling time from the medical center for a minimum of 6 months after transplantation. The candidate's family should be capable of long-term supportive care of the child, who will have exceptional needs.

No clinical suspicion of sepsis should exist. This condition can be confirmed by blood cultures. A normal neurologic evaluation is necessary and can be confirmed by ultrasound, computed tomography scan, and electroencephalogram, if appropriate. Factors that can exclude a potential recipient from heart transplantation include the following:

1. Marked prematurity and low birth weight
2. An unclear cardiac diagnosis
3. Persistent acidosis with pH below 7.10
4. Active sepsis
5. Abnormal neurologic evaluation
6. Abnormal renal function
7. Positive drug screen
8. Significant dysmorphy or genetic problem

Once a recipient is identified, the search for a donor is undertaken.

The first step after identification of a potential organ donor is recognition of clinical signs of brain death. Although exact criteria may vary from state to state, they usually include: lack of response to external stimuli; lack of nonspinal cord reflex activity; lack of brainstem reflexes, including absence of pupillary, corneal, oculocephalic, oculovestibular gag, and cough reflexes. Apnea in the presence of adequate carbon dioxide stimulus is another criterion.

Presence of the required criteria is a signal to summon the professional responsible for brain-death diagnosis. This professional is usually a neurologist, neurosurgeon, or intensive care specialist. It may be desirable in some situations to have a second physician corroborate the findings and to have a confirmatory test, such as an electroencephalogram, performed. Electrocerebral quiescence may confirm brain death, but it is not necessary for declaration of same. The absence of cerebral blood flow, as demonstrated by radio-nuclear isotope studies, can provide near-absolute information in suspected brain death.[19] Although the donor may have required antibiotics, he or she should be clinically free of infection at the time that the heart is procured. Electrocardiogram and echocardiogram should be normal, although mild echocardiographic abnormalities in structure or function may not disqualify a heart from consideration. In general, a left ventricular shortening fraction of greater than 28% is acceptable. Inotropic support and volume resuscitation may be required. Creatine kinase MB isoenzyme level is assessed. Donor ABO type must be compatible with potential recipient, and an appropriate size match is also necessary.

Acceptable renal function is defined as a blood urea nitrogen level below 30 mg/dL and serum creatinine level below 1.5 mg/dL. If either value is greater, a pediatric nephrology consultation is obtained to exclude gross renal abnormalities. The patient should also be phenotypically normal.

CARE OF THE POTENTIAL DONOR

Once brain death has been diagnosed, immediate attention must be given to maintenance of organ function. Prolonged maintenance of a brain-dead individual results in deterioration of organ function primarily as a consequence of decline in systemic perfusion. Adherence to an established donor-monitoring protocol insures that organs are recovered in optimal condition. The following principles are essential to such a protocol:

1. Maintenance of optimal tissue and organ perfusion
2. Maintenance of fluid and electrolyte balance
3. Maintenance of pulmonary function
4. Prevention of infection
5. Maintenance of normal temperature

Hemodynamic management is essential, and hemodynamic status must be meticulously assessed if adequate perfusion of potential donor organs is to be maintained. Inotropic support may not be necessary after fluid loading is accomplished. Development of diabetes insipidus is common in brain-dead organ donors as a result of the failure of the hypothalamus or posterior pituitary gland to produce or release antidiuretic hormone. The result is an abnormally high output of dilute urine, which results in hypovolemia, falling blood pressure, and decreased systemic perfusion. This condition must be treated immediately with fluid replacement and with infusions of vasopressin to maintain blood pressure.

The following documents are necessary from the potential pediatric donor:

1. Parent's consent for organ donation
2. Parent's consent for transport of the body to the appropriate hospital
3. Brain death certificate by two physicians or progress notes that documente brain death and are signed by two physicians, preferably pediatricians
4. Copy of death certificate if the donor is being transported to another facility
5. Documentation of the coroner's consent
6. Consent for cremation, if indicated
7. Copy of the donor chart
8. Copy of chest x-ray, echocardiogram (M-mode and two-dimensional) and electrocardiogram.
9. Blood donor specimens for infectious disease screening and HLA typing

At Loma Linda University Medical Center, the following protocol is used when a donor infant is transferred from another facility to the transplant center:[20]

1. Loma Linda University Medical Center Neonatal Transport Team travels to the donor point of origin. If the donor is to be returned to the Loma Linda University Medical Center, documents needed before initiating donor transport include the following:
   a. Two signatures of brain death, preferably from the pediatric neurologist at the donor point of origin (state laws vary)
   b. Death certificate signed at the donor point of origin, if available
   c. Coroner's consent at the donor point of origin
   d. Family consent for donation, including consent for transport to Loma Linda University Medical Center
   e. Instruction as to handling and return of the body
   f. Permit to return the body if crossing state lines
2. Documents that should be with the donor in transit include the following:

a. Evidence of brain death confirmation
b. Death certificate, if available
c. Coroner's agreement
d. Cardiac diagnostic studies
e. Consent for cremation, if indicated
f. Copy of the donor chart
g. If body is to be returned across state line, permission to embalm and burial certificate are required

The donor is then transported to Loma Linda University Medical Center and admitted to the Neonatal Intensive Care unit. The donor is once again evaluated by a neonatologist, a pediatric neurologist, a pediatric cardiologist, and a pediatric infectious disease specialist. If an infant is found to be a satisfactory donor after this extensive evaluation, supportive care is provided until the time of surgery, when donor and recipient are taken to adjacent operating rooms. Heart procurement is accomplished. Multiple lymph nodes, blood, and spleen are obtained for processing in our immunology labs. Once procurement is complete, the graft is stored in 4°C normal saline (500 mL, to which 10 mL of 50% dextrose has been added).

CARE OF THE POTENTIAL RECIPIENT

A recipient who has met the inclusion criteria for heart transplantation may require continuous intensive care while awaiting donor acquisition and transfer. In cases of hypoplastic left heart syndrome, a continuous PGE_1 infusion by central or peripheral line at dosages of 0.0125 to 0.05 $\mu g/kg/min$ is started. Once the ductus arteriosus is opened, the PGE_1 dose can often be reduced, thereby decreasing unwanted side effects. Infants with this syndrome depend on a patient ductus arteriosus for maintenance of systemic and coronary circulations. Prostaglandin inhibits closure of the ductus and thus allows ejection of blood from the right ventricle into both the pulmonary and systemic circulations.

Blood gases should be kept as close to the stable preoperative state as possible, with oxygen saturations of 65% to 75% and a relatively normal Pco_2. Controlled ventilation is instituted, if necessary, to achieve these goals. Attempts are made to maintain normal blood pressure.

If cardiac inotropic drugs are needed, dopamine is used in doses up to 10 $\mu g/kg/min$. High doses of inotropic drugs may cause undesirable increases in systemic vascular resistance relative to pulmonary vascular resistance, so caution should be used. Diuretics are administered when required to control pulmonary edema.

Appropriate nutritional support is provided. Intragastric tube feedings or parenteral nutritional support is administered, depending on hemodynamic stability and assessment of systemic perfusion. If the recipient's peripheral circulation is marginal, then total parenteral nutrition is instituted.

Transfusion of blood products is avoided. However, if pulmonary resistance and saturations are low, transfusion of washed red blood cells increases oxygen delivery and viscosity, effectively increasing peripheral vascular resistance.

Careful balance of the ratio of pulmonary-to-systemic resistance through manipulation of ventilatory and pharmacologic support is needed because of competition of the parallel circulations. Goals include spontaneous or controlled ventilation with low inspired oxygen concentration, while maintaining Pco_2 above 40 mm Hg. Hypocarbia and hyperoxia are avoided since they decrease pulmonary vascular resistance. A normal newborn maintains a Pco_2 of 40 mm Hg and an arterial oxygen saturation of about 80%. These levels are near the plateau of the fetal oxyhemoglobin dissociation curve and provide adequate oxygen transport to the tissues.

Patients are usually transfused to achieve a hemoglobin of at least 10 g. It is recommended that peripheral intravenous lines be used first, then central lines as a last resort, as low flow states have been noted to result in venous thromboses. Their occurrence can be diminished with this graduated approach to the placement of venous lines.

BLOOD BANK PROTOCOL

Transplant patients have special needs that require more care by the blood bank before products can be given. Preparing blood products may take up to 6 hours after notification of heart transplant surgery. Demands for a shorter turnaround time on all tests depend on the circumstances that surround both the recipient and prospective donor. Once the decision is made that heart transplantation will definitely occur, ABO and Rh typing are completed and appropriate blood products are ordered from the blood bank. These include washed red blood cells, packed red blood cells, platelet concentrate, and fresh frozen plasma. All blood products should be checked for the presence of cytomegalovirus, and only negative units should be used. Blood is tested for histocompatibility (anti-donor antibodies screen). Red cell antibody screening crossmatches are accomplished, and then all blood products are irradiated.[21]

PREANESTHETIC CONSIDERATIONS

The skill with which anesthesia is administered to the recipient is important, as these infants have abnormal cardiorespiratory physiology. Management of this abnormal physiology may differ from that in the neonatal intensive care unit or the pediatric intensive care unit because of the changes in physiology that accompany induction, intubation, mechanical ventilation, and the stress of operation before cardiopulmonary bypass. Deterioration of physiologic status often occurs during the transport to the operating room. Optimum management of the recipient requires communication between the surgeon and the anesthesiologist regarding the underlying anatomy, current physiologic status of the patient, intravenous access, the monitoring of catheters that are in place, the need for ventilatory support, and the current respiratory status. Other considerations include current drug therapy and any additional complications or considerations.

ANESTHETIC MANAGEMENT

Anesthetic management of the neonatal transplant recipient is similar to that of other neonates with congenital heart disease who require surgery accompanied by profound hypothermic circulatory arrest. Management includes the following:

1. Complete operating room equipment set up (Table 2-1).
2. Control of ventilation. Patients who are not intubated preoperatively are intubated and their ventilation controlled in the operating room before placement of any additional monitoring catheters (i.e., percutaneous placement of arterial and central venous pressures).
3. Muscle relaxation. We use pancuronium bromide as the primary muscle relaxant, but vecuronium and atracurium can also be used.
4. Fentanyl citrate anesthesia. Fentanyl citrate is used because of the cardiovascular stability that accompanies its administration in infants, particularly those with hypoplastic left heart syndrome.
5. Hypothermia. Surface cooling is initiated after all catheters and monitors are placed and surgical preparation is started. Heat lamps are turned off, as are heating pads. The head is placed in ice. Core temperature generally drifts to 33° to 35°C before institution of car-

TABLE 2-1. Operating Room Equipment

Monitors

ECG
Noninvasive blood pressure
Pulse oximeter
Stethoscopes: precordial and esophageal
Temperature probes: esophageal, tympanic, rectal
Capnometer
Invasive monitors: arterial and central venous with appropriate insertion kits

IV Set-ups

Peripheral IV
Blood warmer
Manifold line and drug infusion line
Electronic pump for infusion line
Syringe pumps for drug infusions
Selection of catheters for IV access

diopulmonary bypass. Patients are cooled to about 16°C before circulatory arrest, which lasts about 1 hour.

6. Inotropic and vasoactive drugs to aid in separation from cardiopulmonary bypass (Table 2-2).

The possibility of right ventricular failure in the transplanted heart due to elevated pulmonary vascular resistance was a concern when our neonatal heart transplantation program began. Infusions of isoproterenol in combination with dopamine are most commonly used. No sign of

TABLE 2-2. Resuscitation Drugs

Drug	Concentration
Dopamine* Dobutamine Amrinone	1 mL/hr = 5 µg/kg/min
Nitroglycerine Sodium nitroprusside	1 mL/hr = 1 µg/kg/min 1 mL/hr = 0.05 µg/kg/min
Epinephrine Norepinephrine Isoproterenol*	1 mL/hr = 0.05 µg/kg/min
Tolazoline	1 mL/hr = 1 mg/kg/hr

*Most commonly used.

massive right ventricular failure has been noted in our series, and tolaz-oline hydrochloride has not been required.[22] Calcium gluconate is usu-ally the first inotrope used when mean arterial pressure is inadequate and the central venous pressure is high. The decision to use calcium, and inotropes in general, is made by analysis of the heart rate, mean arterial pressure, and central venous pressure, combined with clinical impres-sion of the appearance of the heart. Isoproterenol is used when the heart rate is inadequate and is started at an initial dose of 0.03 μg/kg/min and titrated to achieve a rate of 130 to 150 beats per minute. Dopamine is used to augment isoproterenol when the heart rate is adequate but, also when mean arterial pressure or the appearance of the heart indicates the need for additional inotropic support. Most patients are separated from cardiopulmonary bypass easily and need relatively low doses of vaso-active drugs. All patients have survived the surgical procedure.

Other considerations include blood product treatment and risk of infection, especially in light of immunosuppressive therapy. Blood prod-ucts are irradiated and red blood cells are double-washed before use to reduce the number and slow the metabolism of any active lymphocytes. Blood is also screened for donor antibody, cytomegalovirus, hepatitis, and human immunodeficiency viruses.

The risk of infection in the immunosuppressed patient is the pri-mary factor in the decision not to monitor pulmonary vascular pressures directly. Although technically feasible, clinical results suggest that this step is unnecessary.

Patients have been mechanically ventilated for up to 1 week post-operatively. Vasoactive drugs have been discontinued within 1 week in all long-term survivors.

OPERATIVE METHOD

Surgical technique of cardiac transplantation in neonates and young infants with inoperable congenital heart disease and cardiomyopathy is the same as for adults, with the exception of the use of profound hypo-thermic circulatory arrest. Techniques of transplantation in neonates and young infants with hypoplastic left heart syndrome have been reported and are illustrated and summarized here.[23]

The infant's thorax is opened via midsternal incision, and the peri-cardium is opened in the midline. A near-total thymectomy is per-formed. The aorta and its branches are isolated, and the great vessels are cannulated to establish extracorporeal circulation (Fig. 2-1). A venous cannula is inserted into the right atrium. The arterial cannula is placed

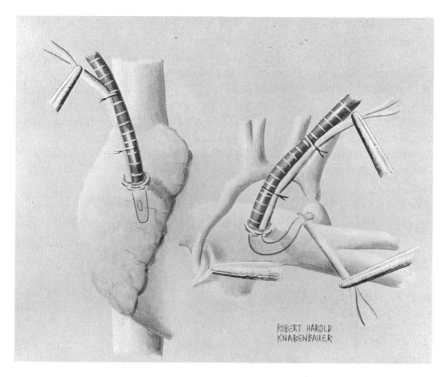

FIGURE 2-1.   Insertion of cannulae for cardiopulmonary bypass. On the left, a venous cannula is inserted into the right atrium. On the right, the arterial cannula is placed through the distal main pulmonary artery into the patent ductus arteriosus.

through the distal main pulmonary artery into the patent ductus arteriosus. Perfusion is established, and a snare is tightened around the ductus that contains the arterial perfusion cannula. The infant is cooled to a core (rectal) temperature near 20°C. The esophageal temperature is16° to 18°C. Aortic arch vessel snares are tightened, perfusion is discontinued, and the patient's blood is emptied into the pump oxygenator. Perfusion cannulae are removed, and the ductus is ligated at its pulmonary artery base.

The heart is excised, with the posterior atrial walls and septum left in place. The main pulmonary artery is transected at its bifurcation into right and left pulmonary arteries. The ascending aorta, which is hypoplastic, is ligated and transected just proximal to the brachiocephalic trunk. The ligated ductus arteriosus is excised from the side of the proximal descending thoracic aorta. The underside of the aortic arch is incised from the level of the brachiocephalic trunk to the ductus excision site and several millimeters beyond (Fig. 2-2).

The donor heart is brought into the pericardial wall and suturing with continuous 7-0 polypropylene is begun with the atrial septum and continued around the right and left atria. The portion of donor aorta distal to the arch vessels is divided squarely, incised on the greater curvature for a length of 20 mm or more (Fig. 2-3), and joined to the opened recipient aorta with a wide anastomosis. The donor pulmonary artery is prepared by excising right and left pulmonary arteries separately and then incising an arterial bridge between. This process provides adequate cir-

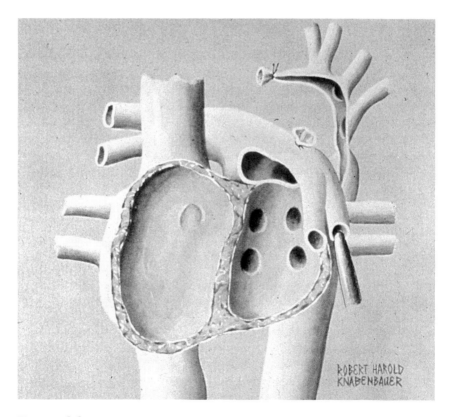

FIGURE 2-2.   Intact recipient posterior atrial walls and septum. The ascending aorta, which is hypoplastic, is ligated and transected just proximal to the brachiocephalic trunk. The ligated ductus arteriosus is excised from the side of the proximal descending thoracic aorta. The underside of the aortic arch is incised from the level of the brachiocephalic trunk to the ductus excision site and slightly beyond.

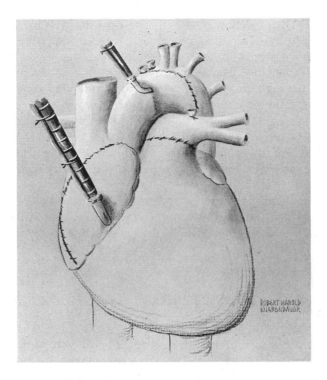

FIGURE 2-3. The donor heart sutured in place.

cumference for anastomosis with the recipient's enlarged distal main pulmonary artery trunk.

The donor heart is intermittently bathed with cold saline (4°C) to insure myocardial preservation. The aorta is filled with cold saline by way of the donor brachiocephalic arterial stump, which is also used for insertion of the arterial cannula for extracorporeal circulation. Purse-string sutures are placed around the tips of both donor atrial appendages. The venous cannula for extracorporeal circulation is inserted into the donor right atrium by way of the purse-string suture in the appendage. The tip of the left arterial appendage is excised to vent the left side of the heart. A needle hole is placed in the ascending aorta as an air vent and cardiopulmonary bypass is reinstituted. The patient is tilted head down to insure that all air is removed from within the cardiovascular chambers, and the arch vessel snares are released. Before separation from cardiopulmonary bypass, temporary pacemaker wires may be attached to the right ventricle and/or right atrium and used as needed.

Heart transplantation after palliative operations, such as systemic-pulmonary shunts, Norwood, or Fontan procedures, is accomplished in much the same way as outlined above. However, the surgical team must consider the need to replace or augment surgically altered structures. The donor harvest team may need to return with extended portions of systemic veins, pulmonary arteries or aorta with which to accomplish the transplantation and reconstruction. Depending on the anticipated ischemic time, the recipient surgical team should be prepared to start dissection long before the expected arrival of the harvest team. As with any reoperation, alternative sites for arterial and venous cannulation should be available.

Finally, retransplantation may become as commonplace in children as it has become in adults. Dissection and replacement of a diseased graft follows well-established principles of reoperation.[24]

PATIENT TRANSPORT FROM THE OPERATING ROOM

Ideally the patient's recovery room is attached directly to the operating room; however, in most hospitals this proximity is not possible. The operating room notifies the intensive care unit when cardiopulmonary bypass is discontinued. At this time, the intensive care unit can make last minute arrangements such as ventilator set-up, various inotropic agents that may be required, and so on. The primary ICU receiving nurse comes to the operating room to help ready the patient for transport. At this time, the anesthesiologist can give the nurse information that will be helpful in the care of the patient postoperatively, and the nurse can also help with the physical transport of the patient.

All patients are transported with continuous electrocardiographic and central venous and systemic blood pressure monitoring. The patient is transported in a warm incubator so that core temperature is maintained. Protective isolation, including mask, gown and 3-minute hand washing, is enforced.

These patients require one-to-one bedside nursing and close respiratory therapy support. The patient is observed for any signs of acute congestive heart failure, hypovolemia, hypothermia, or cardiac arrhythmia. Once the patient is stable, attempts are made to wean from mechanical ventilation as soon as is reasonable.

The patient is also observed for signs of graft rejection, which may clinically be seen as an unexplained persistent increase in resting heart rate, presence of a third heart sound, arrhythmia, tachypnea, diaphoresis, or cool extremities. Irritability, malaise, fever, oliguria, or persistent changes in feeding, sleeping, and other activity patterns may also help diagnose early graft rejection. Rapidly increasing left ventricular posterior and septal wall thickness, decreasing posterior wall and septal systolic and diastolic function, new pericardial effusion, new aortic valve insufficiency, or decreasing left ventricular fiber shortening fraction as demonstrated by echocardiography are all positive indications of early rejection. Other signs of rejection include:

Chest x-ray: advancing global cardiomegaly and pulmonary edema or pleural effusion; Electrocardiogram: reduction in combined voltages greater than or equal to 25%, significant change in QRS axis, arrhythmia (PAC's, PVC's, transient heart block); Laboratory analysis: increasing spontaneous blastogenesis and elevated CPK-MB isoenzyme level.

If the patient has persistent, equivocal signs of rejection, histologic confirmation of rejection is obtained by endomyocardial biopsy.

Since 1973, endomyocardial biopsy has been used successfully to diagnose acute cardiac rejection in adult heart transplant patients. Many noninvasive methods to predict rejection have been tried, but thus far the biopsy method has remained superior. In more than 15,000 biopsies performed at Stanford University in adults, no mortality has been reported and less than 3% morbidity. Of 521 biopsies in 30 children with an age range of 1 month to 15 years, 8 (1.51%) biopsies were inadequate for evaluation and 121 (23.3%) were positive for acute rejection. One biopsy-related death occurred in a 2-month old infant. From this series of patients, it can be concluded that: endomyocardial biopsy can be performed successfully in infants and very young children; the risk in infants younger than 1 year is increased; and biopsy should be performed only when clinically indicated and may not be justified on a routine basis.[25]

IMMUNE REGULATION

The success of any form of transplantation depends on regulating the immune system's response to the transplanted organ. The methods used to achieve such regulation continue to change and vary considerably with the age at which the patient is transplanted. For example, it appears that the immunosuppressive requirements for an infant who receives a heart transplantation during the first month or so of life may be significantly different from infants and children beyond this age group. The exact mechanism for this "graft tolerance" is poorly understood but could be related to persistent maternal–fetal factors that allow immunologic tolerance of the fetus within the mother. The more aggressive immune response experienced among older infants and children may relate to increased exposure to environmental pathogens. Despite these differences, maintenance immunosuppression is essential for achieving continuing graft tolerance.

As soon as a donor is identified, cyclosporine (0.1–0.5 mg/kg/h) is given to the recipient as a continuous intravenous infusion. This infusion is continued postoperatively until the patient is tolerating oral intake. At that point, oral cyclosporine (12–20 mg/kg/day) is started. Trough levels (by monoclonal antibody testing) of 200 to 300 ng/mL are maintained. Trough levels of cyclosporine are tapered over the first year to 100 to 150 ng/mL. These levels have correlated with excellent graft tolerance and with minimal, if any, hypertension or renal impairment.

Intravenous azathioprine (3 mg/kg) is given daily perioperatively. This dose is adjusted to keep the white blood cell count greater than 4000/mm^3. It is changed to the same oral dose after the patient begins eating and is continued for at least the first postoperative year. In those children who were older than 1 month of age when they received their transplantation, it has been Loma Linda policy to taper dosage but continue azathioprine indefinitely . Azathioprine is discontinued after the first year for neonatal transplant recipients.

Despite adequate levels of maintenance immunosuppression, rejection can and does occur in most infant and child transplant recipients. Rejection episodes are more frequent in older infants and children, such that additional agents are currently under evaluation as induction therapy to reduce or potentially eliminate rejection (Table 2-3). Although highly successful in some adult transplant centers, OKT3, a monoclonal antibody directed against a specific T-cell lymphocyte subgroup, has been less effective in the pediatric age group. Recent Loma Linda experience with Vanderbilt rabbit antithymocyte serum (ATS) has been gratifying. Its efficacy as induction therapy in older infants is currently being evaluated by randomized trials.

Rejection episodes that cannot be prevented are treated according to their severity. Rejection episodes in infants, particularly neonates, are usually mild and can be treated on an outpatient basis with intravenous steroids, using more frequent daily surveillance until resolved. Symptomatic rejection episodes are handled on an inpatient basis with 125 mg of methylprednisolone twice daily for six to eight doses. Rejection that responds slowly to intravenous steroids, has produced hemodynamic compromise, or that does not respond appropriately to two courses of intravenous steroids is treated additionally with ATS or occasionally

TABLE 2-3. Rejection Protocol

Symptoms	Treatment
Asymptomatic, minimal	Methylprednisolone 125 mg every 12 h IV for 3–4 days in outpatient setting
Moderate to severe	Inpatient IV steroid (as above); and/or antithymocyte serum 0.5 mL/kg/day IV for 7–10 days *in intensive care setting;* Extracorporeal membrane oxygenation, optional rescue therapy
If recipient is older than 30 days when transplanted, female, with a poor HLA match and receiving a male heart	IV methylprednisolone at time of rejection diagnosis; if indications for rejection not reversed within 24 hours, begin immediately:
	Antithymocyte serum, pretreat with benadryl 1 mg/kg IV (perhaps more useful in infants or children); or OKT$_3$ 3–5 mg IV for 5–10 days; pretreat with benadryl; IV or oral steroid administration should continue; Tylenol elixir or suppository in dose appropriate for age

with methotrexate. Rarely, hemodynamic decompensation is so sudden or intense that temporary extracorporeal circulation is required for several days to allow the antirejection drugs to take effect.

Infection of the transplanted recipient is a potentially lethal complication and has accounted for a significant percent of early and late mortality among older children and adults. Incidence of lethal infection may well reflect the more intense immune suppression used in most centers for these older recipients. Infection, although quite common, has been an unusual cause of death after pediatric heart transplantation in the Loma Linda experience, perhaps because immunosuppressive maintenance dose is considerably less for the younger age group. Moreover, the absence of routine steroid therapy may contribute to the extremely low incidence of serious infection in these patients. Recipients with infections are managed with appropriate antimicrobial agents. Cytomegalovirus infection is so ubiquitous among immunosuppressed patients that Loma Linda current protocol includes routine prophylactic use of gamma globulin infusions (400–600 mg/kg/day) perioperatively and acyclovir (20–30 mg/kg/day) orally during the first 3 postoperative months. Patients with symptomatic cytomegalovirus infection are given a 2-week course of intravenous gancyclovir (3–5 mg/kg/day) and supplemental gamma globulin.

Most of the common childhood immunizations, including diphtheria, pertussis, tetanus, polio (Salk), pneumococcus, hemophilus influenza B, and influenza A and B, are administered. However, vaccination for measles, mumps, and rubella are deferred, owing to the live viruses involved. Opportunistic infection and infestations with such organisms as *Pneumocystis carinii*, *Nocardia* species, *Mycobacterium* species, and fungus have been unusual among pediatric recipients whose immune modulation follows the protocol described above.

COMPLICATIONS

The twin threats of graft rejection and host infection, which together account for the majority of early and late deaths after heart transplantation, have already been mentioned. Other complications are listed in Table 2-4.

Systemic hypertension complicates post-transplant treatment in virtually every adult patient and, despite the aggressive use of various combinations of diuretics, vasodilators, and sympatholytic drugs, remains a difficult problem to manage. Experience in children has been mixed. The

TABLE 2-4.   Complications of Pediatric Heart Transplantation (Loma Linda University)

System	Complications
Renal	Acute or chronic failure
Gastrointestinal	Gastroesophageal reflux
	Feeding disorders
	Peptide ulceration
Neurologic	Seizures
	Cerebrovascular accident
Pulmonary	Pneumonia
	Atelectasis
	Bronchospasm
	Pleural effusion
	Pulmonary vascular hypertensive crisis
Integumentary	Hirsutism
	Gingival hyperplasia
Cardiovascular	Rejection
	Graft failure without rejection
	Hypertension
	Residual or recurrent aortic coarctation
	Bradyarrhythmia

Stanford University group reported significant hypertension in 96% of their pediatric population.[24] At the University of Pittsburgh, hypertension was present in more than half of the long-term survivors.[25] At Loma Linda, few survivors have required chronic antihypertensive treatment. We feel this fact is due to an individualized, minimal immunosuppressive regimen.

Renal dysfunction is the most common and troublesome adverse effect of chronic cyclosporine therapy after heart transplantation in adults.[26] In children, a plasma creatinine rise to a mean level of 2 mg/dL was observed at 2 years by the Stanford group, without further deterioration between 2 and 4 years.[24] Several institutions have reported normal late renal function.[25,27,28] At Loma Linda University, some patients had perioperative renal dysfunction, but any recipient who was severely oliguric or anuric perioperatively was aggressively treated with peritoneal dialysis.[29] Few survivors have shown evidence of chronic renal dysfunction.

Coronary artery disease (CAD) represents the main impediment to long-term survival of adult heart transplant patients, since it has been the major complication responsible for graft failures in both the precyclosporine and cyclosporine eras.[2,30] The Harefield Hospital group reported no CAD in 57 children with heart or heart–lung transplantation after a mean follow-up of 21 months.[31] The longest follow-up of a newborn heart transplant recipient in the Loma Linda series is more than 5 years, and that patient has no evidence of atherosclerosis on a recent coronary angiogram. Interestingly, both the Harefield and the Loma Linda groups avoid chronic steroid immunosuppression in the pediatric population because of concern that steroids accelerate CAD.

Malignancy is more common in transplanted patients as a consequence of impairment of intrinsic host immunosurveillance, direct action of immunosuppressive drugs, chronic antigenic stimulation by the allograft, and activation of oncogenic viruses. The incidence of lymphoproliferative disorders, usually non-Hodgkin's lymphoma, is less than 1%.[26]

CONCLUSION

Currently, 10% of all cardiac transplantations annually are performed in the pediatric age group. This percentage will increase, since the annual number of adult cardiac transplantations has leveled off in the past 4 years while the number of pediatric recipients continues to rise.

At Loma Linda University, 107 pediatric patients younger than 12 years of age were transplanted between 1985 and 1990. Operative mortality (less than 30 postoperative days) was 13%. However, in 1990, 33 of 35 patients (96%) survived the operation. Older infants and children experience a similar early mortality rate, but late mortality appears to be higher. Actuarial survival associated with pediatric cardiac transplantation is 82% at 1 year and 67% at 5 years. The neonatal subgroup has a 1-year survival of 87% and a 5-year survival of 84%.

Treatment of several congenital heart anomalies with cardiac transplantation appears to provide a more favorable prognosis than that achieved with palliative operations, as 5-year survival does not compare with that which is possible with cardiac transplantation.

Recent advances in transplant immunotherapy appear extremely promising, and more effective post-transplant immunosuppression will further expand the indications for heart transplantation.

References

1. Schroeder JS, Hunt SA: Cardiac transplantation: Update 1987. JAMA 258:3142, 1987
2. Pennock JL, Oyer PE, Reitz BA et al: Cardiac transplantation in perspective for the future: Survival, complications, rehabilitation, and cost. J Thorac Cardiovasc Surg 83:168, 1982
3. Goodwin JF: Cardiac transplantation. Circulation 74:913, 1986
4. Lough ME, Lindsey AM, Shinn JA et al: Life satisfaction following heart transplantation. J Heart Transplant 4:446, 1985
5. Samuelsson RG, Hunt SA, Schroeder JS: Functional and social rehabilitation of heart transplant recipients under age thirty. Scand J Thorac Cardiovasc Surg 18:97, 1984
6. Christopherson LK, Griepp RB, Stinson EF: Rehabilitation after cardiac transplantation. JAMA 326:2082, 1976
7. Stevenson LW, Fowler MB, Schroeder JS, Stevenson WG, Dracup KA, Fond V: Poor survival of patients with idiopathic cardiomyopathy considered too well for transplantation. Am J Med 83:871, 1987
8. Oyer PE, Stinson EB, Reitz BA et al: Cardiac transplantation: 1980. Transplant Proc 13:199, 1981
9. Packer M: Prolonging life in patients with congestive heart failure: The next frontier. Circulation (suppl IV)75:1, 1987
10. Kaye MP: The Registry of the International Society for Heart Transplantation: Fourth Official Report, 1987. J Heart Transplant 6:63, 1987
11. Penkoske PA, Rowe RD, Freedom RM et al: The future of heart and heart–lung transplantation in children. Heart Transplantation 3:233, 1984
12. Addonizio LJ, Rose EA: Cardiac transplantation in children and adolescents. J Pediatr 111:1034, 1987
13. Pennington DG, Sarafian J, Swartz M: Heart transplantation in children. Heart Transplantation 4:441, 1985
14. Dunn JM, Cavarocchi NC, Balsara RK et al: Pediatric heart transplantation at St. Christopher's Hospital for Children. J Heart Transplant 6:334, 1987

15. Kantrowitz A, Haller JD, Joos H, Cerruti MM, Carstensen HE: Transplantation of the heart in an infant and an adult. Am J Cardiol 22:782, 1968
16. Cooley DA, Bloodwell Rd, Hallman GL, Nora JJ, Harrison GM: Organ transplantation for advanced cardiopulmonary disease. Ann Thorac Surg 8:30, 1969
17. Bailey LL, Nehlsen-Cannarella SI, Concepcion W, Jolley WB: Baboon to human cardiac xenotransplantation in a neonate. JAMA 254:3321, 1985
18. Loma Linda International Heart Institute Infant Heart Transplantation Protocol, 1990.
19. Drake B, Ashwal S, Schneider S: Determination of cerebral death in the pediatric intensive care unit. Pediatrics 78:107, 1986
20. Martin RD, Parisi F, Robinson TW, Bailey LL: Anesthetic management of neonatal cardiac transplantation. J Cardiothoracic Anesthesia 3:465, 1989
21. Bailey LL, Concepcion W, Shattuck H, Huang L: Method of heart transplantation for treatment of hypoplastic left heart syndrome. J Thoracic Cardiac Surg 92:1, 1986
22. Chiavarelli M, De Begona JA, Vigesaa RE et al: Heart transplantation in children. Advances in Cardiac Surgery 3 (in press)
23. Billingham M: The gold standard: Endomyocardial biopsy (abstr). Presented at the Loma Linda International Conference on Pediatric Heart Transplantation, March 1990. Loma Linda, CA.
24. Starnes VA, Stinson EB, Oyer PE et al: Cardiac transplantation in children and adolescents. Circulation 76(suppl V):43, 1987
25. Pahl E, Fricker J, Armitage J et al: Coronary arteriosclerosis in pediatric heart transplant survivors: Limitation of long-term survival. J Pediatr 116:177, 1990
26. Kahan BD: Immunosuppressive therapy with cyclosporine for cardiac transplantation. Circulation 75:40, 1987
27. Addonizio LJ, Hsu DT, Smith CR, Gersony WM, Rose EA: Late complications in pediatric cardiac transplant recipients. Circulation 82(suppl IV):295, 1990
28. Chartrand C, Dumont L, Stanley P: Pediatric cardiac transplantation. Transplant Proc 21:3349, 1989
29. Vricella L, Alonso de Begona J, Gundry S et al: Agressive peritoneal dialysis for treatment of renal failure after neonatal cardiac transplant. Presented at the International Society for Heart Transplantation, 11th Annual Meeting and Scientific Sessions, Paris, France, April 1991
30. Uretsky BF, Murali S, Reddy PS et al: Development of coronary artery disease in cardiac transplant patients receiving immunosuppressive therapy with cyclosporine and prednisone. Circulation 76:827, 1987
31. Radley-Smith R, Yacoub MF: Heart and heart-lung transplantation in children. Circulation 76(suppl IV):24, 1987

Marc D. Thames
Carol M. Buchter

New Insights Into Cardiovascular Physiology Obtained After Cardiac

3 Transplantation

Before cardiac transplantation, patients usually have severe congestive heart failure and markedly impaired cardiac function. Under these circumstances, autonomic control of the heart and circulation is impaired, and the reflex mechanisms that normally regulate sympathetic and parasympathetic outflow to the heart and peripheral circulation are markedly abnormal.[1-3] After cardiac transplantation, heart failure is reversed and cardiac function is normalized. However, additional changes that occur may be important in the regulation of the cardiovascular system. For example, interruption of efferent sympathetic and parasympathetic nerves to the donor organ occurs, affecting the myocardium, the conduction system, and the coronary arteries. In addition, sensory fibers that originate from chemosensitive and mechanosensitive endings in the ventricles, particularly the left ventricle, are interrupted by cardiac transplantation. After surgery is completed, immunosuppressive agents are used to control rejection. Rejection has important effects on the donor organ, particularly on the myocardium and the coronary arteries. Finally, as the survival of patients with cardiac transplantation continues to improve, the possibility of reinnervation of the transplanted heart may become an increasingly important consideration. Thus, the transplant model provides a unique opportunity to study a variety of different aspects of cardiovascular regulation and function. It is the purpose of this brief review to summarize some of the new insights into cardiovascular regulation that have been obtained from patients with cardiac transplantation, with a specific emphasis on the effects of deefferentation and deafferentation, reversal of heart failure, and reinnervation.

EFFECTS OF CARDIAC DEEFFERENTATION

Effects of Parasympathetic Deefferentation

The parasympathetic nerves that travel in the cervical vagi are preganglionic fibers. These fibers synapse with postganglionic fibers that originate from ganglion cells in the heart. Interruption of preganglionic neurons results in loss of control of the postganglionic fibers, even when the latter are transplanted with the donor heart. The result is probably best illustrated by the loss of vagal effects on the transplanted sinus node.[4,5] In normal subjects, respiration-related variability of the R-R interval occurs, called respiratory sinus arrhythmia. This sinus arrhythmia is particularly prominent in dogs and has been shown to be abolished after cardiac autotransplantation.[6] Patients with heart failure have low resting vagal tone and little sinus arrhythmia. In human subjects studied up to 5 years after cardiac transplantation, minimal variation in the R-R interval of the denervated donor heart is seen with respiration, and this fact does not change with the passage of time.[5,7] On the other hand, the respiration-related changes in cycle length of the innervated recipient atrium (P-P interval) return toward normal values after transplantation and reversal of heart failure. Figure 3-1 illustrates the effect of transplantation on recipient atrium and donor cardiac cycle length and contrasts these data with those obtained in patients with heart failure or in subjects who have no cardiac disease. It has been shown by a number of investigators that the cardiac deefferentation associated with cardiac transplantation abolishes vagal effects on the atrioventricular (AV) node as well as on the sinus node.

Effects on cardiac electrophysiology also have been studied. Denervation of the sinus and AV nodes has been shown to convey supersensitivity to the effects of acetylcholine in a canine model.[8] The endogenous metabolite adenosine and the neurotransmitter acetylcholine have similar electrophysiologic effects on the sinus and AV nodes that are mediated by a common transduction process. Ellenbogen and colleagues recently studied the effects of adenosine on the innervated and denervated sinus node and the denervated AV node of patients after cardiac transplantation to determine if denervation conveys hypersensitive responses to adenosine.[9] The effects of adenosine on sinus cycle length

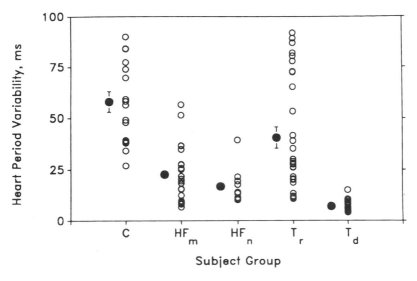

FIGURE 3-1. Heart period variability measured during quiet rest in 16 healthy control subjects *(C)*, 23 medicated patients with heart failure (*HF*$_m$), 11 nonmedicated patients with heart failure (*HF*$_n$), 21 donor atria of orthotopic cardiac transplant patients (T$_d$), and 30 recipient atria of orthotopic cardiac transplant patients (*T*$_r$). Each open circle represents an individual subject, whereas the solid circles and brackets represent the group means ± standard error of the mean. The transplant recipient heart period variability was not significantly different from the control group but was significantly different from that of the donor hearts. Note that congestive heart failure resulted in significant impairment of heart period variability. *(Smith ML, Ellenbogen KA, Eckberg DL, Szentpetery S, Thames MD: Reversal of abnormal parasympathetic control of heart period following cardiac transplantation. J Am Coll Cardiol 14:106, 1989)*

of the innervated recipient atrium and of the donor denervated atrium are illustrated in Figure 3-2. Denervation resulted in supersensitive responses to adenosine. Supersensitive responses of the AV node also were demonstrated. These supersensitive responses to adenosine may help to explain episodes of marked sinus bradycardia that occur during acute severe cardiac rejection. Ellenbogen and colleagues have demonstrated that administration of low-dose theophylline, an agent that antagonizes the effects of adenosine on the sinus and AV nodes, is effective in reversing this bradycardia.[10] It is possible that the supersensitivity that was detected in these studies is the result of up-regulation or increased availability of the G protein that is coupled to the adenosine A1 receptor and may be shared by muscarinic cholinergic mechanisms.

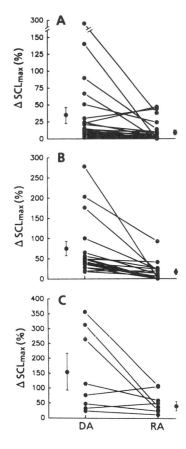

FIGURE 3-2. Scatter plots illustrate changes in sinus cycle length (Δ SCL$_{max}$, %) for individual donor and recipient atria in transplant patients after incremental doses of adenosine. DA, donor denervated atrial electrogram; RA, recipient innervated atrial electrogram. Responses illustrated in A, B, and C are for increasing doses of adenosine (37, 75, and 112 µg/kg injected over 3 to 5 seconds). Note differences in scale for ordinate in the three graphs. *(Ellenbogen KA, Thames MD, DiMarco JP, Sheehan HM, Lerman BB: Electrophysiological effects of adenosine on the transplanted human heart: Evidence of Supersensitivity. Circulation 81:821, 1990)*

Effects of Sympathetic Deefferentation

Interruption of sympathetic nerves to the heart interrupts sympathetic innervation of the myocardium, the conduction system, and the coronary arteries. Initially, great concern was expressed regarding the potentially negative effects that this interruption might have on exercise performance. However, it was shown subsequently that the cardiac responses of animals and humans with cardiac denervation are largely preserved as a result of increases in heart rate and contractility due to increases in circulating catecholamines and to Frank Starling mechanisms early in exercise before significant tachycardia has occurred.[11] Elimination of the circulating catecholamines by β-adrenergic blockade impairs maximal exercise responses in dogs with cardiac denervation[11] and humans with cardiac transplantation, thus indicating the importance of circulating catecholamines in supporting the denervated heart at high levels of exercise.

Cardiac transplantation interrupts the sympathetic innervation of the coronary circulation. Hodgson and colleagues recently investigated the relative contribution of α- and β-adrenergic mechanisms to the control of resting coronary vascular resistance in patients after transplantation.[12] They found that α-receptor-mediated vascular tone is modest in both denervated transplant patients and normally innervated patients; however, increases in vascular resistance observed after β-adrenergic blockade are due principally to withdrawal of β-adrenergic tone in normally innervated patients and to unopposed α-constrictor tone in patients with cardiac transplantation. β-Adrenergic vasodilation was found to be mediated by β_2-adrenergic receptor stimulation. The major findings of their study are illustrated in Figure 3-3.

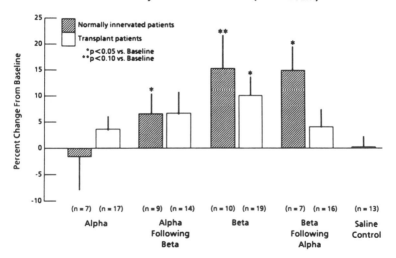

FIGURE 3-3.   Coronary vascular resistance index after specific receptor blockade for both normally innervated (crosshatched bars) and transplant (open bars) patients. Note that β-adrenergic blockade increased coronary vascular resistance significantly before, but not after, α-adrenergic blockade. (Hodgson JMcB, Cohen MD, Szentpetery S, Thames MD: Effects of regional alpha- and beta-blockage on resting and hyperemic coronary blood flow in conscious, unstressed humans with cardiac denervation. Circulation 79:797, 1989)

Coronary denervation may alter vascular reactivity. Bertrand and colleagues reported that cardiac autotransplantation was used to treat coronary vasospasm that was causing Prinzmetal's angina in a 49-year-old man with anatomically normal coronary arteries.[13] Complete cardiac denervation did not prevent ergonovine-induced coronary vasospasm but was successful in abolishing spontaneous episodes of spasm. It also abolished the sensation of angina during ergonovine-induced coronary artery spasm, thereby establishing the cardiac source of his chest pain.

EFFECTS OF CARDIAC DEAFFERENTATION

When the heart is transplanted, the recipient's atrial remnant, which retains most of the atrial sensory receptors, is left in place. Little is known about the function of these atrial receptors. On the other hand, the donor organ, which normally is richly innervated by sensory receptors in the ventricles, becomes deafferented. Two kinds of sensory mechanisms exist in the ventricles, particularly in the left ventricle. One is a mechanoreceptor, which responds to changes in cardiac mechanics and pressures, while the other is a chemosensitive ending, which responds to chemical agents such as prostaglandins and radiographic contrast.[14]

Mechanoreflexes

In normal subjects, application of negative pressure to the lower part of the body results in pooling of blood in the lower extremities and reflex vasoconstriction.[15] Animal studies indicate that these responses are most likely mediated by sensory receptors in the cardiopulmonary region.[14] Reducing the filling of the heart reduces the discharge of these mechanoreceptors, resulting in the withdrawal of their tonic inhibitory influence on sympathetic outflow to the heart and circulation. This disinhibition results in sympathoexcitation. Recent experimental data suggest that sensory receptors in the left ventricle may be especially important in mediating reflex vasoconstrictor responses to lower body negative pressure (LBNP).[16] This stimulus is the functional equivalent of a hemorrhage in the sense that the blood is redistributed from the central circulation to the veins of the legs and, thus, has the same effect on the central circulation as hemorrhage or orthostatic stress. Mohanty and colleagues have reported that, after cardiac transplantation and reversal of the heart failure, the responses to LBNP are impaired (Fig. 3-4).[16] This result is not from a nonspecific impairment of reflex control, since the response of

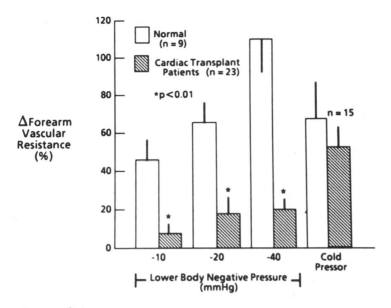

FIGURE 3-4.   Changes in forearm vascular resistance (%) to LBNP and cold pressor test in nine normal subjects (open bars) and in 23 cardiac transplant patients (crosshatched bars). Cold pressor response was assessed in 15 of the 23 cardiac transplant patients. Significant differences between normal subjects and cardiac transplant patients are so indicated. LBNP was performed at three levels of suction, including −10, −20, and −40 mm Hg. Note that the responses to LBNP in the transplant patients are markedly impaired. (Mohanty PK, Thames MD, Sowers JR, McNamara C, Szentpetery S: Impairment of cardiopulmonary barosreflex following cardiac transplantation in humans. Circulation 75:914, 1987)

these subjects to the cold pressor test is normal, and, as outlined below, the arterial baroreflex control of the innervated recipient sinus node becomes normal after transplantation. It also is not the result of the effects of immunosuppressive therapy, since patients with renal transplantation have preserved responses to LBNP. Preliminary data from Victor and colleagues have been interpreted to indicate that reflex responses to LBNP are preserved after cardiac transplantation.[17] They measured muscle sympathetic nerve activity rather than forearm vascular resistance. Unfortunately, decreases in arterial pressure occurred during LBNP in their study, whereas no significant decreases in arterial blood pressure occurred during lower body suction in the study by Mohanty and colleagues.[16] Thus, in the latter study, the stimulus was relatively selective for sensory receptors in the cardiopulmonary region, while in the former study clear effects on arterial baroreflexes could have accounted for the observed responses.

Chemoreflexes

In addition to the mechanosensitive receptors, cardiac sensory C fibers respond to a variety of irritant substances, including meglumine diatrizoate, a commonly used radiographic contrast agent.[13] When this agent is administered by intracoronary injection, it results in reflex bradycardia and hypotension. If the receptors responsible for these reflex changes are located throughout the heart, then we would predict some preservation of these responses, even after cardiac transplantation, since the recipient atria retain their innervation. Arrowood and colleagues have reported that the bradycardia and hypotension that normally result from intracoronary injection of meglumine diatrizoate are abolished after cardiac transplantation.[18] In fact, they showed that the nontransplanted portion of the heart exhibits reflex *tachycardia* because of the hypotension that results from contrast injection. They also demonstrated direct effects of contrast on the denervated donor sinus node. This chemoreflex has previously been called the Bezold-Jarisch reflex, and the data of Arrowood and colleagues indicate that the sensory receptors responsible for this reflex are located entirely in the transplanted portion of the heart.[18] Since the atrial remnant retains its innervation, both afferent and efferent, these data suggest that the ventricles are the exclusive location for the sensory receptors that mediate this response.

Vasovagal Syncope

It has been proposed that during vasovagal syncope, such as occurs while standing for prolonged periods in hot environments, venous pooling in the lower extremities results in hypotension and reflex sympathoexcitation. This condition results in marked inotropic stimulation of the heart at low filling pressures and, thereby, in markedly increased intramyocardial distortional forces that would increase the activity of mechanosensitive endings in the left ventricle. These endings normally respond to increases in cardiac filling pressure. This paradoxical activation of mechanoreceptors at low filling pressures would restore their tonic inhibitory influence on sympathetic nerve activity and promote vasodilation.[19] It would also augment the excitatory influence of these endings on vagal outflow to the heart. A recent important observation from Scherrer and colleagues suggests that this mechanism may not be the cause of vasovagal syncope.[20] They infused nitroprusside into a patient with a transplanted heart and recorded the electrocardiogram and muscle sympathetic nerve activity in this subject. On termination of the nitroprusside infusion, the patient began to feel as if he were passing out, and the investigators observed, despite a falling arterial pressure, slowing of the recipient's innervated sinus node and inhibition of muscle sympathetic nerve activity occurred. This response closely mimics the autonomic response to vasovagal syncope, suggesting that ventricular receptors are not necessary for the induction of vasovagal syncope and that some other mechanism should be considered as the principal cause of this important clinical syndrome.

EFFECTS OF REVERSAL OF HEART FAILURE

Effects on Arterial Baroreflexes

It is well known that arterial baroreflex control of heart rate (or R-R interval) is markedly abnormal in animals and humans with congestive heart failure.[21] Treatment of heart failure with medications has been shown to improve this abnormality, but the extent of improvement is modest. Ellenbogen and colleagues reported that arterial baroreflex control of the innervated recipient sinus node (P-P interval) becomes normal after cardiac transplantation (Fig. 3-5).[4] In fact, they observed this normalization as early as several days after the operation. Since most of the baroreflex-mediated slowing of the heart rate or prolongation of the heart interval is mediated by increased parasympathetic outflow to the sinus node, these data indicate that parasympathetic control of the sinus node recovers rapidly after cardiac transplantation and normalization of cardiac function. This rapid recovery is important because it suggests that these abnormalities are not due to underlying structural changes in the heart or the sensory receptors themselves but are more likely due to neuro-humoral abnormalities that alter reflex control.

Effects on Resting Vagal Tone

As noted above, marked recovery of the resting vagal tone of the recipient-innervated sinus node occurs after cardiac transplantation.[5,7] This recovery is an indication of restoration of resting parasympathetic tone

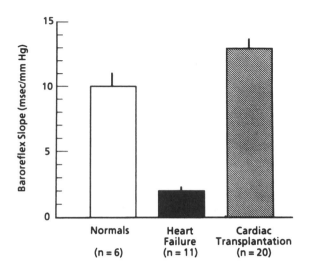

FIGURE 3-5.   Bar graph of baroreflex slopes
(baroreflex sensitivities) in control subjects (open bars),
heart failure patients (solid bars) and in patients with
cardiac transplantation (crosshatched bars). A
statistically significant difference was found between
the mean baroreflex sensitivity for the heart failure
patients compared with control subjects and
transplant patients. No significant difference was seen
between the baroreflex slope in control patients and
transplant patients. These data indicate complete
recovery of the baroreflex control of the innervated
recipient sinus node after transplantation and reversal
of heart failure. *(Ellenbogen KA, Mohanty PK,
Szentpetery S, Thames MD: Baroreflex abnormalities in
heart failure: Reversal after orthotopic cardiac
transplantation. Circulation 79:51, 1989)*

to the sinus node, which is markedly reduced in congestive heart failure.
The extent to which the recovery of this resting vagal tone occurs is
related to age and blood pressure, since many patients with cardiac
transplantation treated with cyclosporine have some degree of hypertension that also reduces resting vagal tone and thus recipient sinus node P-
P interval variability.

REINNERVATION OF THE TRANSPLANTED HEART

Animal Studies

It has been known for some time that the autotransplanted canine heart is rapidly reinnervated with both sympathetic and parasympathetic efferent nerves. Parasympathetic reinnervation occurs generally in the first 3 to 4 months, while sympathetic reinnervation occurs during the first year. This reinnervation has been shown to be functionally important and may even occur in some animals with cardiac homotransplantation that are on immunosuppression. Mohanty and colleagues have reported that dogs subjected to cardiac autotransplantation still have some reduction in myocardial catecholamine levels compared to normal controls after 8 to 12 years.[21] Mohanty and colleagues also found afferent reinnervation of the heart in these dogs with long-term cardiac autotransplantation.[22] They found that responses to stimulation of left ventricular receptors with left ventricular injection of veratrum alkaloids in dogs with cardiac transplantation were still modestly impaired even up to 12 years after transplantation. However, marked recovery of this reflex response occurred (Fig. 3-6), indicating that afferent reinnervation of the transplanted heart could occur in the long term. Earlier studies in dogs indicated that such afferent reinnervation was unusual during the first 2 years after cardiac transplantation.[23]

Human Studies

As the effectiveness of immunosuppressive therapy increases and the survival of patients with cardiac transplantation is prolonged, the possibility that reinnervation of the transplanted human heart may occur is considered by some to be highly probable. To date, no evidence for functional parasympathetic reinnervation of the donor heart exists. Ellenbogen and colleagues studied the responses of patients with cardiac transplantation to the intravenous administration of phenylephrine up to 4 years after transplantation and detected no baroreflex slowing of the donor sinus node in these subjects.[4] Smith and colleagues, as noted above, found no evidence of recovery of heart period variability up to 4 years after transplantation.[5,7] P-P interval variability was used as an index of resting vagal tone to the sinus node. Thus, there is little reason to believe that functional parasympathetic reinnervation of the donor denervated heart occurs.

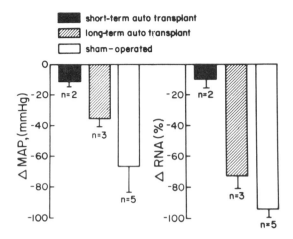

△ MAP(mmHg) and △ RNA(%) Following
LV Cryptenamine

FIGURE 3-6. Responses of renal nerve activity
(Δ RNA [%]) and mean arterial pressure (MAP) to
chemical stimulation of cardiac receptors with left
ventricular injection of cryptenamine (a veratrum
alkaloid mixture) in sham-operated dogs (open bars)
and dogs with cardiac autotransplantation. The
markedly impaired response in the group with
short-term autotransplantation (closed bars)
suggests afferent denervation, whereas a greater
response in the group with long-term
autotransplantation (crosshatched bars) suggests
afferent reinnervation of the heart. *(Mohanty PK,
Thames MD, Capehart JR, Kawaguchi A, Ballon B,
Lower RR: Afferent reinnervation of the
autotransplanted heart in dogs. J Am Coll Cardiol
7:419, 1986)*

In contrast to this persistence of parasympathetic denervation,
recent evidence suggests that sympathetic reinnervation of the denervated donor organ may occur. Schweiger and colleagues used positron
emission tomographic methods and [11C] hydroxyephedrine to demonstrate that the anterobasal and superior septal areas of the transplanted donor heart developed some efferent sympathetic reinnervation
3 and a half years after transplantation.[24] The more apical regions of the

heart remained devoid of innervation. Wilson and colleagues have detected norepinephrine release from the donor heart after intracoronary administration of tyramine, a finding that is also consistent with some sympathetic reinnervation.[25] Two biopsy studies provide conflicting evidence regarding the presence of sympathetic reinnervation of the donor heart.[26,27] Some caution should be used in considering the importance of the presence of some sympathetic reinnervation and its ability to respond to tyramine, as, to date, no evidence of functionally significant sympathetic reinnervation of the heart exists.

CONCLUSION

After cardiac transplantation, congestive heart failure is reduced and afferent and efferent cardiac nerve fibers are interrupted. Over the course of time, some sympathetic reinnervation may occur, but its functional significance is uncertain. The heart transplant patient provides an interesting model for studying the mechanisms of cardiovascular regulation and has helped us to obtain new insights into the control of the conduction system, cardiac function, and the coronary arteries. It is anticipated that continued investigations along these lines will provide new insights into mechanisms of cardiovascular regulation.

References

1. Dibner-Dunlap ME, Thames MD: Abnormalities of baroreflex control in heart failure. Heart Failure 6:12, 1990
2. Ferguson DW: Baroreflex-mediated circulatory control in human heart failure. Heart Failure 6:3, 1990
3. Zucker IH, Wang W, Chen J-S: Baroreceptor and cardiac receptor abnormalities in experimental heart failure. Heart Failure 6:17, 1990
4. Ellenbogen KA, Mohanty PK, Szentpetery S, Thames MD: Baroreflex abnormalities in heart failure: Reversal after orthotopic cardiac transplantation. Circulation 79:51, 1989
5. Smith ML, Ellenbogen KA, Eckberg DL, Szentpetery S, Thames MD: Reversal of abnormal parasympathetic control of heart period following cardiac transplantation. J Am Coll Cardiol 14:106, 1989
6. Thames MD, Kontos HA, Lower RR: Sinus arrhythmia in dogs after cardiac transplantation. Am J Cardiol 24:54, 1969
7. Smith ML, Ellenbogen KA, Eckberg DL, Sheehan HM, Thames MD: Subnormal parasympathetic activity after cardiac transplantation. Am J Cardiol 66:1243, 1990
8. Minardo JD, Tuli MM, Mock BH et al: Scintigraphic and electrophysiological evidence of canine myocardial sympathetic denervation and reinner-

vation produced by myocardial infarction or phenol application. Circulation 78:1008, 1988

9. Ellenbogen KA, Thames MD, DiMarco JP, Sheehan HM, Lerman BB: Electrophysiological effects of adenosine on the transplanted human heart: Evidence of supersensitivity. Circulation 81:821, 1990

10. Ellenbogen KA, Szentpetery S, Katz MR: Reversibility of prolonged chronotropic dysfunction with theophylline following orthotopic cardiac transplantation. Am Heart J 116:202, 1988

11. Donald DE, Shepherd JT: Initial cardiovascular adjustment to exercise in dogs with chronic cardiac denervation. Am J Physiol 207:1325, 1964

12. Hodgson JMcB, Cohen MD, Szentpetery S, Thames MD: Effects of regional alpha- and beta-blockade on resting and hyperemic coronary blood flow in conscious, unstressed humans with cardiac denervation. Circulation 79:797, 1989

13. Bertrand ME, Lablanche JM, Tilmant PY, Ducloux G, Warembourg H, Soots G: Complete denervation of the heart (autotransplantation) for treatment of severe, refractory coronary spasm. Am J Cardiol 47:1375, 1981

14. Minisi AJ, Thames MD: Reflexes from ventricular receptors with vagal afferents. In Zucker IH, Gilmore JP (eds): Reflex Control of the Circulation, p. 359. Boca Raton, CRC Press, 1991

15. Zoller RP, Mark AL, Abbolud FM et al: The role of low pressure baroreceptors in reflex vasoconstrictor responses in man. J Clin Invest 51:2967, 1972

16. Mohanty PK, Thames MD, Sowers JR, McNamara C, Szentpetery S: Impairment of cardiopulmonary baroreflex following cardiac transplantation in humans. Circulation 75:914, 1987

17. Victor R, Scherrer U, Vissing S, Morgan B, Urias L. Hansen P: Orthostatic stress activates sympathetic outflow in patient with heart transplants (abstr). Circulation 78:II-365, 1988

18. Arrowood JA, Mohanty PK, Hodgson JMcB, Dibner-Dunlap ME, Thames MD: Ventricular sensory endings mediate reflex bradycardia during coronary arteriography in humans. Circulation 80:1293, 1989

19. Thoren P: Role of cardiac vagal C-fibers in cardiovascular control. Rev Physiol Biochem Pharmacol 86:1, 1979

20. Scherrer U, Vissing S, Morgan B, Hansen P, Victor R: Vasovagal syncope after infusion of a vasodilator in a heart transplant recipient. N Engl J Med 322:602, 1990

21. Mohanty PK, Sowers JR, Thames MD, Beck FWJ, Kawaguchi A, Lower RR: Myocardial norepinephrine, epinephrine and dopamine concentrations after cardiac autotransplantation in dogs. J Am Coll Cardiol 7:414, 1986

22. Mohanty PK, Thames MD, Capehart JR, Kawaguchi A, Ballon B, Lower RR: Afferent reinnervation of the autotransplanted heart in dogs. J Am Coll Cardiol 7:419, 1986

23. Thames MD, Zubair-ul-Hassan, Brackett NC Jr, Lower RR, Kontos HA: Plasma renin responses to hemorrhage after cardiac autotransplantation. Am J Physiol 221:1115, 1971

24. Schweiger M, Hutchins G, Kalff V et al: Evidence for regional catecholamine uptake and storage sites in the transplanted heart by positron emission tomography. J Clin Invest 87:1681, 1991

25. Wilson R, Christensen B, Simon A, Olivari MT, White C: Evidence for struc-

tural sympathetic reinnervation after cardiac transplantation in humans. Circulation (in press) 83:1210, 1991

26. Bristow M: The surgically denervated, transplanted human heart. Circulation 82:658, 1990

27. Regitz V, Bossaller C, Strasser R, Schuler S, Hetzer R, Fleck E: Myocardial catecholamine content after heart transplantation. Circulation 82:620, 1990

Kane M. High
Walter E. Pae, Jr.
Frederick A. Hensley, Jr

Mechanical Support as a Bridge to Cardiac

4 | Transplantation

RESULTS OF MECHANICAL CIRCULATORY SUPPORT

It is well appreciated that 20% of all candidates for cardiac transplantation die before a donor organ is obtained.[1] The encouraging results obtained with temporary mechanical ventricular assistance in patients with postcardiotomy cardiogenic shock have led to the use of this modality in conjunction with cardiac transplantation.[2] Experiences with aggressive mechanical circulatory support in conjunction with transplantation have been limited to reports in the medical literature that describe rather small institutional experiences with multiple devices. Multicenter clinical trials with established protocols have been lacking. Therefore, it has been difficult to assess immediate outcome, compare device effectiveness, and examine overall impact on availability of donor organs and ultimate long-term survival.

More recently, in an attempt to overcome this lack of information, data have been collected by the Combined Registry for the clinical use of ventricular assist pumps and the total artificial heart (TAH) sponsored by the International Society for Heart Transplantation and the American Society for Artificial Internal Organs.[2,3] This large computerized data base has allowed for comparison of clinical results, and the following describes information submitted to the Combined Registry since its inception in 1985.

Indications for circulatory support followed by heart transplantation fit into two broad categories: (1) acute rejection with hemodynamic deterioration after transplantation, and (2) hemodynamic deterioration before orthotopic heart transplantation. The first group comprises a relatively small number of patients. As of December 31, 1989, 37 patients reported to the Combined Registry had acute rejection after transplantation and required circulatory support. Of these, 22 (9%) were successfully supported with mechanical assistance and underwent second transplant procedures, and 7 (32%) of the 22 were ultimately discharged from the hospital. This absolute salvage rate of 19% is discouraging. The second, and larger, group of patients consists of those awaiting transplantation who require hemodynamic support because of donor organ unavailability. In this group of 363 patients reported to the Registry, 83% were males with a mean age of 43, paralleling the normal transplant population demographics, as expected.

The wide range of duration of circulatory support necessary until the patient's condition stabilizes or a donor organ becomes available underscores the necessity for devices that provide safe and reliable short, intermediate, and long-term support. Support was provided for 18.0 ± 0.1 days (0–439) (mean ± SEM, range) in all patients reported. Of this total, support was provided for 19.9 ± 4.4 (0–396) days in patients not transplanted, 17.3 ± 2.3 (0–439) days in all patients who were transplanted, and 15.0 ± 1.7 (0–137) daysin those who were transplanted and discharged from the hospital.

The overall results of staged heart transplantation (i.e., circulatory support followed by transplantation) are summarized in Table 4-1. In the 400 patients who received ventricular assistance, the number of days of circulatory support based on the type of device appears to show a significant difference between ventricular assist devices (VAD) and the TAH, with shorter durations found with the VADs. This finding may be due to anticipation of longer support intervals in patients with problems such as unusual blood types, high antibody levels, higher incidences of medical complications that require longer support before transplantation, or other patient selection criteria. Univentricular support was provided to 89 patients (22% of all patients), 130 received biventricular support (33% of all patients), and 178 received the TAH (45% of all patients). Rates of subsequent transplantation were similar irrespective of the type of support used: 67% for left ventricular assist devices (LVAD), 64% for biventricular assist devices (BVAD) and 72% for the TAH. However, the hospital discharge rate was significantly different between the groups, with the lowest rate displayed in those patients with the TAH (47%), and the best rate with the LVAD alone (80%; p < 0.01

TABLE 4-1. Overall Results of Bridge to Transplantation as of
December 31, 1989

System	Number of Patients	Number of Days mean ± SEM**	Transplanted (%)	Discharged (%)
LVAD	89	16.6 ± 0.3 (0–153)	60 (67.4)	48 (80.0)
RVAD	3	2.0 ± 1.1 (0–5)	1 (33.3)	1 (100.0)
BVAD	130	11.0 ± 0.1 (0–83)	83 (63.8)	54 (65.1)
TAH	178	24.0 ± 0.3*	128 (71.9)	60 (46.9)†
Total	400	(0–439)	272 (68.0)	163 (59.9)

LVAD, left ventricular assist device; RVAD, right ventricular assist device; BVAD, biventricular assist device; TAH, total artificial heart.

*$P < 0.01$, Student-Newman-Keuls test, TAH vs. BVAD and TAH vs. LVAD.

†$P < 0.01$ by chi-squared analysis.

**P Standard error of the mean.

(Modified from Miller CA, Pae WE Jr, Pierce WS: Combined Registry for the clinical use of mechanical ventricular assist pumps and the total artificial heart in conjunction with heart transplantation: Fourth official report, 1989. J Heart Transplant 9:453, 1990)

by chi-squared analysis).[4] This difference is probably related to the longer support times, as well as the previously mentioned issues. It is interesting that the rates of subsequent transplantation and hospital discharge were independent of the type of ventricular assist pump used, whether pneumatic, centrifugal, or electric powered[4] (Table 4-2).

The 2-year actuarial survival curve for all types of circulatory support in patients who underwent staged orthotopic heart transplantation

TABLE 4-2. Overall Outcome of Staged Heart Transplantation
Based on the Type of Ventricular Assist Pump

Type	Number of Patients	Transplant (%)	Discharged (%)
Pneumatic (excluding TAH)	127	87 (68.5)	63 (72.4)
Centrifugal	50	28 (56.0)	19 (67.9)
Electric	41	22 (53.7)	19 (86.4)

TAH, total artificial heart.

(Miller CA, Pae WE Jr, Pierce WS: Combined Registry for the clinical use of mechanical ventricular assist pumps and the total artificial heart in conjunction with heart transplantation: Fourth official report, 1989. J Heart Transplant 9:453, 1990)

is demonstrated in Figure 4-1. The Kaplan-Meier survival rate at 2 years is 65%, which is in contrast to the near 80% survival of patients who undergo isolated orthotopic heart transplantation.[3] Nevertheless, when survival estimates are prepared for each type of mechanical support, the patients who receive univentricular support approach the same actuarial survival rate as the general heart transplant population (Fig. 4-2). A significant difference is apparent in ultimate survival based on the type of device used, with univentricular support having the most favorable results and the TAH having the least favorable ($P < 0.0001$).

The complications that preclude a subsequent heart transplant procedure are shown in Table 4-3. Obviously, many patients had more than one complication. Step-wise logistic regression analysis indicates that renal failure, biventricular failure, and respiratory failure (in order of decreasing importance) had a significant negative impact on future

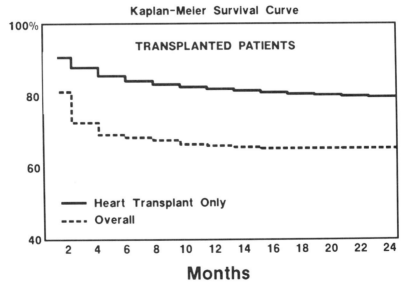

FIGURE 4-1.   Kaplan-Meier actual 2-year survival curve. Survival of staged heart transplantation as compared to transplant only. The survival rate at 2 years is 65% for staged transplants in contrast to the near 80% survival of patients who undergo isolated orthotopic heart transplantation. (*Miller CA, Pae WE Jr, Pierce WS: Combined Registry for the clinical use of mechanical ventricular assist pumps and the total artificial heart in conjunction with heart transplantation: Fourth official report, 1989. J Heart Transplant 9:453, 1990*)

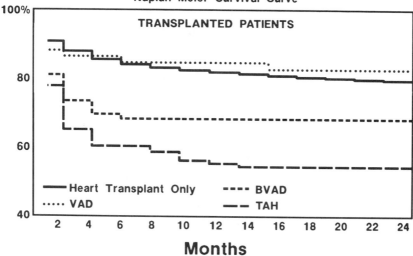

STAGED CARDIAC TRANSPLANTATION
Kaplan-Meier Survival Curve

TRANSPLANTED PATIENTS

— Heart Transplant Only   ---- BVAD
····· VAD   — — TAH

Months

FIGURE 4-2. Kaplan-Meier actuarial 2-year survival based on the type of support and compared to transplant only. Single *VAD* survival at 2 years similar to isolated orthotopic heart transplantation but decreased for *BVAD* and *TAH*. *(Miller CA, Pae WE Jr, Pierce WS: Combined Registry for the clinical use of mechanical ventricular assist pumps and the total artificial heart in conjunction with heart transplantation: Fourth official report, 1989. J Heart Transplant 9:453, 1990)*

TABLE 4-3. Complications That Precluded Transplantation for All Years

Complication	Total (n = 128) (%)	VAD (n = 31) (%)	BVAD (n = 47) (%)	TAH (n = 50) (%)
Infection	20	23	13	24
Biventricular failure	24	45	36	NA
Kidney failure	27	23	13	40*
Respiratory failure	26	19	17	38*
Central nervous system death	14	16	17	10
Bleeding	20	23	21	18
Multiorgan failure	12	0	4	26†

VAD, ventricular assist device; BVAD, biventricular assist device; TAH, total artificial heart; NA, not applicable.
*P <0.05 by Fisher's exact test, BVAD vs. TAH.
†P <0.05 by Fisher's exact test, BVAD vs. TAH and VAD vs. TAH.
(Miller CA, Pae WE Jr, Pierce WS: Combined Registry for the clinical use of mechanical ventricular assist pumps and the total artificial heart in conjunction with heart transplantation: Fourth official report, 1989. J Heart Transplant 9:453, 1990)

transplantation. Fishers exact test suggested that those patients bridged with a TAH had a significantly higher rate of multiorgan failure, precluding subsequent transplant, than those patients supported with univentricular or biventricular devices ($P < 0.05$). Total artificial heart recipients also had a 40% rate of renal failure, which was significantly higher than the 15% rate seen in patients supported with the paracorporeal BVAD ($P < 0.05$).[4]

Table 4-4 illustrates the causes of death after transplantation with each type of ventricular assistance. Again, any given patient may have had more than one etiologic factor. Other than the fact that those patients previously bridged to transplantation with univentricular assistance had a higher incidence of bleeding (33%) than biventricular (7%) or TAH (9%) patients ($P < 0.05$), complications were similar among the groups.[4] Etiology of increased bleeding in those patients who underwent univentricular support, as compared with the other groups, is not clear. The causes of death at less than or greater than 30 days after transplantation are shown in Table 4-5. Once again, logistic regression analysis indicates that renal failure, infection, and bleeding were the most important predictors of hospital death immediately after heart transplantation. Causes of death after 30 days seemed to parallel those in the general transplant population, with infection and rejection responsible for most deaths.[4]

TABLE 4-4. Causes of Death After Staged Heart Transplantation Based on the Type of Ventricular Assistance

Cause of Death	VAD (n = 12) (%)	BVAD (n = 29) (%)	TAH (n = 68) (%)
Infection	33	21	27
Transplant rejection	0	3	24
Biventricular failure	25	28	7
Bleeding	33*	7	9
Kidney failure	33	14	13
Respiratory failure	25	10	10
Central nervous system death/multiple organ failure	0	10	16
Graft failure	0	14	4

VAD, ventricular assist device; *BVAD*, biventricular assist device; *TAH*, total artificial heart.
*$P < 0.05$ by Fisher's exact test, VAD vs. BVAD and VAD vs. TAH.
(Miller CA, Pae WE Jr, Pierce WS: Combined Registry for the clinical use of mechanical ventricular assist pumps and the total artificial heart in conjunction with heart transplantation: Fourth official report, 1989. J Heart Transplant 9:453, 1990)

TABLE 4-5. Causes of Death After Staged Heart Transplantation

Cause of Death	Less Than 30-Day Mortality (%)	30-Day Mortality (%)
Total applicable patients	75/272	34/272
Infection	28	21
Transplant rejection	13	24
Biventricular failure	19	6
Bleeding	16	0
Kidney failure	15	9
Respiratory failure	15	9
Central nervous system death/multiple organ failure	13	15
Graft failure	9	
Unknown	12	38
Medical noncompliant		6

(Miller CA, Pae WE Jr, Pierce WS: Combined Registry for the clinical use of mechanical ventricular assist pumps and the total artificial heart in conjunction with heart transplantation: Fourth official report, 1989. J Heart Transplant 9:453, 1990)

TYPES OF ASSIST PUMPS

Mechanical assist devices can be classified as pneumatic, electric, or centrifugal pumps. The assist pumps used today are placed outside the chest wall (paracorporeal) or in the upper abdomen and supply blood flow via transcutaneous or transdiaphragmatic cannulae. A general discussion of the operation of each type of pump is undertaken in addition to a more detailed look at a typical or commonly used pump in each group.

Pneumatic

The pneumatic pump shown in Figure 4-3A functions by virtue of blood sacs that have external pressure applied by gas during ejection to force blood into the aorta. Direction of blood flow is controlled by prosthetic valves, which operate as they would in the natural ventricle to prevent reverse flow.[4A]

During systole, the blood sac is squeezed by increased gas pressure within the pump case. During diastole, the pump case is maintained at a negative gauge-pressure, causing blood to be drawn into the pump. The pressures that drive the pumps are generated by a drive unit that is connected to the ventricles by air lines, or "drive lines." The drive unit con-

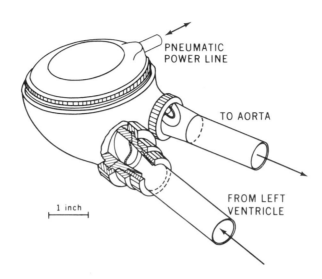

FIGURE 4-3A. Pierce/Donachy pneumatic assist pump. A flexible sac inside a rigid case. Drive line attachment allows air to squeeze the bag, causing ejection out of the pump. Diastolic vacuum causes the bag to re expand with blood entering through the inlet valve. *(High KM, Pierce WS, Skeehan TM: Circulatory assist devices. In Hensley, FA, Martin DE (eds): The Practice of Cardiac Anesthesia, p. 650. Boston, Little, Brown, 1990)*

tains positive pressure (systolic) and negative pressure (diastolic) drive tanks that are alternately connected to the drive lines via a spool valve.

The most commonly used pneumatic assist pumps are versions of the Pierce/Donachy pump commercially produced by Sarns/3M, Inc. (Ann Arbor, MI) and Thoratec Laboratories Corporation (Berkeley, CA). The Pierce/Donachy pump has a maximum stroke volume of 70 mL and a maximum cardiac index of about 7 l/min.

Electric

The Novacor LVAD (Figure 4-3B) is a pusher-plate pump manufactured by Novacor, Inc. (Oakland, CA).[6] It uses plates rather than gas to compress the blood bag. Solenoid valves bend beam springs that are then released to press on the pusher plates and the blood sac. Bioprosthetic valves insure unidirectional blood flow.[7] The device can only be used as a left ventricular assist pump because of its reliance on the generation of adequate ventricular pressure for its own diastolic filling. Apical ventric-

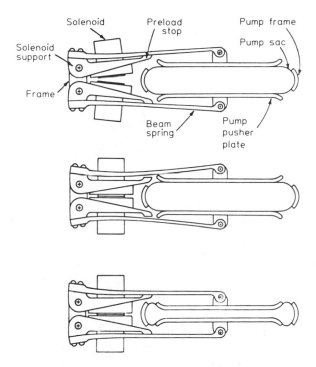

FIGURE 4-3B.   Novacor pusher plate pump. A metal plate squeezes the bag, causing ejection. The pump is shown in the end-diastolic position (top), onset of systole (middle), and end-systolic position (bottom). *(Portner PM, Oyer PE, Jassawalla JS, et al: A totally implantable ventricular assist device for end-stage heart disease. In Unger F (ed): Assisted Circulation 2, p. 122. Heidelberg, Springer-Verlag, 1984)*

ular cannulation limits usefulness in postcardiotomy cardiogenic shock because of damage to an already-compromised ventricle, possible thrombus formation in the ventricle if the cannula is allowed to remain in situ after weaning the pump, and technical difficulties in removing the cannula from the ventricle after the pump is weaned. Obviously, these limits do not apply in the patient being bridged to transplantation.

Centrifugal

Centrifugal pumps (Fig. 4-3C) cause a rotational acceleration of the blood by a spinning impeller powered by an electric motor.[8] The pressure generated by the centrifugal pump is determined by the rotational speed of the blood, the radius of the pump, and density of the fluid (blood).

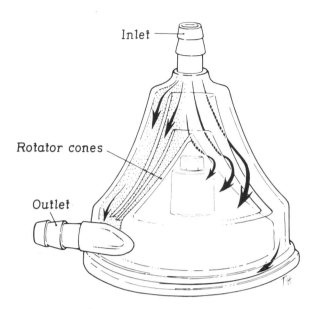

Inlet

Rotator cones

Outlet

FIGURE 4-3C.   Bio Medicus centrifugal pump. A spinning impeller causes the centrifugal acceleration of blood. Blood enters near the axis of the pump and exits at the periphery. *(Reed CC, Stafford TB, (eds): Cardiopulmonary Bypass, 2nd ed, p. 378. Houston, Texas Medical Press, 1985)*

Several important clinical differences between this type of pump and the pneumatic and electric pumps exist. The centrifugal pump has the following:

Nonpulsatile flow: Because the impeller turns at a constant rate, the resultant pressure produced is constant and nonpulsatile. Although debate over the physiologic consequences, exists several long-term studies of metabolic and biochemical parameters have shown that this type of perfusion probably does not cause any deleterious sequelae.

Nonocclusive venous inflow: Whether the centrifugal pump is used for left or right heart assistance, flow through the pump is maintained by the pressure gradient created by the pump. No valves are required in this type of pump because of the continuous forward flow.

Two manufacturers provide centrifugal pumps: Sarns and Bio-Medicus. The BioPump by BioMedicus is used as part of a portable assist system (CPS, by Bard) for support after acute cardiac decompensation. Sarns manufactures the Delphin centrifugal pump.

As shown in Figure 4-4, left ventricular assist pumps generally have their outflow cannulae placed in the ascending aorta. Inflow cannula placement is more variable and can be in the left atrium or left ventricle. Cannulae traverse the diaphragm and exit the skin below the costal margin for the Pierce/Donachy pump, or through the diaphragm to a pre-peritoneal pocket as with the Novacor pump. The inflow cannula for the Pierce/Donachy pump can be inserted into either the atrium or the ventricle, whereas the inlet cannula for the Novacor LVAD must be placed

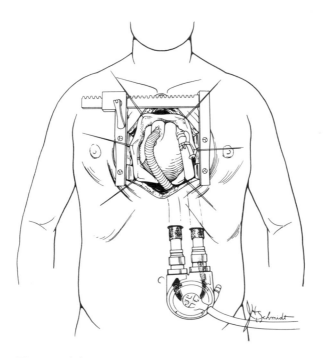

FIGURE 4-4. Positioning of pneumatic LVAD in patient. The inlet and outlet cannulae traverse the diaphragm and pass through the skin in the upper abdomen. In this situation, blood is withdrawn from the left atrium into the pump and is ejected into the aorta. By positioning the inlet cannula in the right atrium and ejecting blood into the pulmonary artery, the device can be used as a RVAD. In the case of biventricular failure, two devices are used. (*High KM, Pierce WS, Skeehan TM: Circulatory assist devices. In Hensley FA, Martin DE (eds): The Practice of Cardiac Anesthesia, p. 653. Boston, Little, Brown, 1990*)

in the left ventricle because of the pump's dependence on left ventricular ejection for filling.

With centrifugal pumps, somewhat longer cannulae traverse the chest wall, and usually the pump is fixed to the patient's bed. The outflow cannula of a right ventricular assist device (RVAD) is connected to the pulmonary artery and the inflow cannula to the right atrium. It functions in an analogous manner to the LVAD. Meticulous de-airing of the cannulae and pump is performed before these pumps are activated.

CONTROL AND OPERATIONS OF ASSIST PUMPS

Pneumatic

Initially, the pump is controlled by changing the pumping rate and driving pressures on the drive unit by hand (manual mode). In the manual mode, a pump rate is set, and the pump may or may not be filling and emptying completely. Once the patient has been weaned from cardiopulmonary bypass and is stable, the pump rate is usually controlled automatically. In the automatic mode, the Pierce/Donachy VAD varies its beat rate so it fills and empties completely with each beat (the "full-to-empty mode") asynchronously with the native heart. This mode of operation provides good washing of the blood sac and inhibits formation of thrombus. Ventricular filling is detected by a Hall-effect switch, and emptying is determined by monitoring the drive line pressure trace for the "empty flag" as shown in Figure 4-5. This "flag" represents a time when gas flow out of the VAD has stopped and the pneumatic drive line pressure has come into equilibrium with the drive unit pressure tanks.

Systolic and diastolic driving pressures can also be adjusted to improve pump performance. They are adjusted to provide full-to-empty pumping while maintaining a desired pump output. The systolic duration can also be adjusted to vary filling and emptying. The pneumatic devices can also be run in a counterpulsation mode, that is, synchronous with the cardiac cycle, but this mode is usually not used because no advantage to it has been shown: the pump no longer runs full to empty, and arrhythmia or a rapid heart rate complicates synchronization.

Electric

Unlike pneumatic pumps, the Novacor pump is usually synchronized to the cardiac cycle and pumps during the diastolic portion. This synchronization is accomplished through two methods: detection of the R wave

LEFT POWER LINE EVENTS

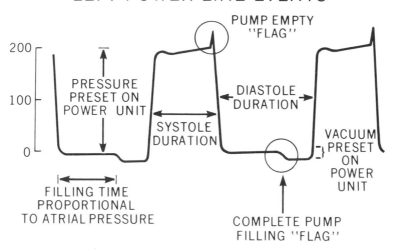

FIGURE 4-5.   Air drive line pressure tracing, "empty flag." At the end of pneumatic pump systole, a short period of no pump ejection can occur. During this period no volume change in the gas in the rigid pump case occurs, and the pressure in the case and the drive line come into equilibrium with the pressure in the systolic drive tank in the drive unit. This event causes at first a pressure increase and then a steady period of pressure called an "empty flag" because it signals emptying of the pump. (High KM, Pierce WS, Skeehan TM: *Circulatory assist devices*. In Hensley FA, Martin DE (eds): *The Practice of Cardiac Anesthesia*, p. 655. Boston, Little, Brown, 1990)

of the electrocardiogram or detection of the end of native ventricular ejection into the pump. End of ejection of the native ventricle is detected as the end of motion of the pusher plate. Thus, this pump does not necessarily fill and empty each stroke; stroke volume varies, depending primarily on the rate of pump filling.

Centrifugal Pumps

Pump speed is manually adjusted so that the pump maintains adequate flow and pressure on its outflow side, while effecting adequate decompression on its inflow or venous side. Thus, for left heart assistance, left atrial pressure would need to be kept below an acceptable maximum value, while the mean arterial pressure would be maintained at an acceptable minimum value. For right heart assistance, central venous pressure would be kept below a safe maximum, while mean pulmonary pressure or left atrial pressure would need to be kept at a reasonable minimum value. These levels are accomplished by adjusting the pump speed and blood volume. However, centrifugal pumps, unlike most pulsatile pumps, can have a reduced pump output in the face of elevated systemic afterload. Therefore, continuous monitoring of pump output is critical.

A summary of the operation and control aspects of assist pumps is given in Table 4-6. As is indicated, the response of pneumatic and electric pumps to increased preload depends on the end-diastolic volume of these pumps before the preload is increased. That is, if these pumps are not completely filling at end-diastole, then the increase of filling pressure increases filling and forward flow. With centrifugal pumps, the increase of preload causes a small increase in output.

Little change is found in the output of the pneumatic and electric pumps in response to changes in afterload. Centrifugal pumps have a moderate decrease in output as afterload increases.

ANTICOAGULATION DURING ASSIST PUMPING

The use of anticoagulants during assist pumping is not a totally resolved issue. Risk of bleeding must be weighed against risk of thrombus formation. As a general rule, regular ventricular contraction, in addition to the use of anticoagulants, helps reduce the risk of clot formation within the native ventricle.

Pneumatic and Electric

Some form of anticoagulation or antiplatelet therapy is generally used for patients with an intact coagulation system. Heparin is the drug usually employed in a dose sufficient to increase the activated clotting time to 150 to 250 seconds. Because of the often short time period between availability of a donor heart and transplantation, low molecular weight dextran is not used, as the prolonged half-life may cause unacceptable coagulopathy. For prolonged mechanical support, patients are anticoagulated with coumadin.

Centrifugal

Studies have been done with and without systemic heparinization, maintaining activated clotting time at a level that ranges from normal control (100 seconds) to about 200 seconds. However, the data are incon-

TABLE 4-6. Comparison of Operation and Control of Assist Pumps

Pump	Mode of Operation	Pump Controlled Variables	Response to Increased Preload	Response to Increased Afterload
Pneumatic				
Pierce/Donachy Thoratec VAD				
Manual	Variable filling	Rate S & D drive pressures S duration	Increased output if increased SV	Little
Automatic	Full-to-empty	S & D drive pressures S duration	Increased rate, thus increased output	Little
Electric				
Novacor	Variable filling synchronized with cardiac cycle	None	Increased filling, thus SV and increased output	Little
Centrifugal				
Bio-Pump	Continous rotation	Speed of rotation	Increased output	Moderate decreased output proportional to increased afterload

VAD, ventricular assist device; S & D, systolic & diastolic; SV, stroke volume; S, systolic.
(*Modified from High KM, Pierce WS, Skeehan TM: Circulatory assist devices. In Hensley FA, Martin DE (eds): The Practice of Cardiac Anesthesia, p 642. Boston, Little Brown, 1990*)

clusive and medical judgment should be used. If bleeding is minimal, some level of anticoagulation is advisable when centrifugal pumps are used. In the future, covalent binding of heparin to pump surfaces may allow the use of this and other pumps without systemic heparinization.

COMPLICATIONS AND LIMITATIONS

The incidence of complications reported in the Combined Registry was discussed earlier in this chapter. However, it is important to consider a few specific points in regard to the operation of assist devices.

Right Ventricular Failure

Many patients who have been supported until transplantation with the LVAD have marginal right ventricular function. Sometimes when the LVAD is applied, right heart failure ensues; it can sometimes be corrected by the concomitant use of inotropes and vasodilators. Generally, right ventricular failure is considered to include a cardiac index less than 1.8 L/min/m^2, with left atrial pressure less than or equal to 15mm Hg and right atrial pressure greater than or equal to 25mm Hg.

A second assist device may be needed for simultaneous right ventricular support. Accurate measurement of left atrial pressure, central venous pressure and cardiac output is necessary to make proper therapeutic decisions regarding not only the need for a right ventricular assist device (RVAD) but also the determination of LVAD pump function, such as the preload required for adequate LVAD output.

Danger of Diastolic Vacuum

Probe Patent Foramen Ovale

This anatomical variation occurs in about 25% of the population and can cause severe intracardiac shunting if left atrial pressure is reduced below right atrial pressure with the aid of diastolic vacuum or suction from a centrifugal pump. Accordingly, the foramen should always be checked and surgically closed at the time of insertion of the left ventricle assist cannulae, if possible.

Open Chest

Diastolic vacuum applied to pneumatic devices during diastole may draw air into the circulation before closure of the chest. Similarly, the negative inflow pressure that can be generated by centrifugal pumps has the potential to draw air into the circulation at suture lines. Risk of air entrainment can be reduced by maintaining adequate filling pressures.

Infection

The large diameter tubes that pass transcutaneously through the chest wall present a serious risk of infection. Despite vigorous attention to wound care at the cannula sites and the use of velour sleeves to allow tissue ingrowth, risk of infection persists throughout the time an assist pump is used. Prophylactic antibiotics are usually used. Once infection is present in these devices, it can almost never be eradicated. Although cardiac transplantation in an infected patient carries considerable risk because of the use of immunosuppressive agents, successful outcomes have been reported in spite of this complication.

Coagulation

Risk of thrombus formation or excessive bleeding is present whenever assist devices are used. The particular risk in any one patient depends on the amount of anticoagulants used. Thrombus formation, although rare, can occur and present a constant risk to the patient. During the perioperative period, risk of hemorrhage is ever-present, particularly along the suture lines that attach the pump cannulae to the patient.

Inflow Occlusion

Obstruction to flow into assist pumps continues to be a concern. Either thrombus formation inside the cannula or extrinsic compression of the cannula or atrium by clot or tissue can prevent adequate flow of blood into the pump. Proper inflow cannula position can be determined by intraoperative use of transesophageal echocardiography in addition to the measurement of the filling pressures and pump flow.[9,10]

Pulsatile vs. Non-pulsatile

As indicated by statistics from the Combined Registry and from other studies, no complications appear to be specific to the use of pulsatile vs. centrifugal pumps for ventricular assistance.[2,3,11-14] Theoretical disadvantages of nonpulsatile flow have not been substantiated. If some form of pulsatile flow is desired with a centrifugal pump, it can be combined with an intra-aortic balloon pump to produce a pulse pressure.

TOTAL ARTIFICIAL HEART

The use of the TAH (Fig. 4-6) to physically and functionally replace the native heart continues in selected patients as a bridge to transplantation.[15,16] Use of the TAH may be considered in patients with severe

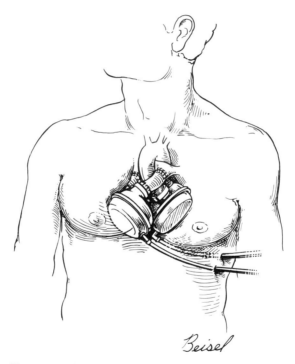

Beisel

FIGURE 4-6.   Surgical placement of the Pennsylvania state TAH. Sewing rings are sutured to the atrial cuffs that were created when the recipient heart was excised. Dacron grafts are attached to the pulmonary artery and aorta. These four connectors are attached to the appropriate ports on the two pumps. (*High KM, Pierce WS, Skeehan TM: Circulatory assist devices. In Hensley FA, Martin DE (eds): The Practice of Cardiac Anesthesia, p. 658. Boston, Little, Brown, 1990*)

biventricular failure with acute rejection or with rupture of the ventricular septum if the patient has adequate chest size. Excision of the native heart is similar to that performed for transplantation. The pneumatic TAH appears similar to two VADs. However, changes have been made in the angulation of the inlet and outlet ports to accommodate the great arteries and veins. Control of the pumping of the TAH is based on analysis of the drive-line pressure waveform that was discussed earlier in this chapter. Because of the apparently higher incidence of complications with the TAH and poorer outcome (see Table 4-3) enthusiasm for its use is diminishing.

ANESTHETIC CONSIDERATIONS

Anesthetic management requires an understanding of how the pumps are being used, how they function, and how they are controlled. In addition, it is necessary to consider the right ventricle and the pulmonary circulation separately from the left ventricle and the systemic circulation. Effects of anesthetics on unassisted ventricles must be considered.

In general, management rules are the following:

1. *Maintain adequate preload.* Anesthetics often cause vasodilation, reducing central blood volume and limiting the ability of the assist device to fill. In patients with a pulsatile VAD, it is desirable not to use vacuum during diastole while the chest is open so that the risk of air entrainment is reduced. Therefore, it is necessary to maintain adequate blood volume to permit the VAD to fill. At the same time, it is necessary not to overload the patient and precipitate ventricular failure to the unassisted ventricle.
2. *Inotropes are often required for the ventricle that is not supported with an assist device.* Vasodilators may help improve output from the unassisted ventricle. Effects of every drug must be considered in terms of the pulmonary and systemic circulations and the unassisted ventricle.
3. *The effects of ventilation on the circulation must be considered.* In a patient with an LVAD in place, mechanical ventilation needs to be managed according to its effects on pulmonary vascular resistance. A high mean airway pressure may increase this resistance. On the other hand, hyperventilation may reduce reactive pulmonary vascular resistance.
4. *Maintaining good communication* with the individual who is controlling the assist device helps ensure that it is functioning appropriately and may help optimize functioning of the assist device.

Total blood flow to the systemic circulation is the sum of the output of the natural ventricle plus that of the LVAD. If no significant native ventricular ejection exists, that is, if the arterial waveform does not have native ventricular pulsations, systemic flow may be calculated as that of the assist pump output alone. For pulsatile pumps, this amount is calculated by multiplying the VAD pump rate by the stroke volume (known if the device is pumping in a full-to-empty mode). If the arterial wave form does show native ventricular pulses, thermodilution cardiac outputs are valid measures of total systemic blood flow. Centrifugal pumps require flow meters to measure pump output. Either electromagnetic flow meters or Doppler flow meters can be used for this purpose.

The use of a RVAD makes determination of systemic blood flow more difficult. Thermodilution cardiac outputs cannot be reliably used because of differing transit times of blood through the RVAD and the native right ventricle. Estimates of RVAD output can be made if the stroke volume of RVAD (full-to-empty mode) and rate are known. Again, this amount is the total cardiac output if the native ventricle is not ejecting. If the native right ventricle is ejecting, total systemic flow can only be determined by the dilutional method using indocyanine green dye. Dye is injected into the pulmonary artery or left atrium, and its concentration is determined in a peripheral (radial) artery.

Output of a Pennsylvania State TAH can be determined from the stroke volume (full-to-empty) and rate of pumping. The TAH output can also be determined with a dilutional method using green dye. Thermodilution cardiac outputs are not readily done because a pulmonary artery catheter should not be placed through the prosthetic valves.

All standard anesthesia monitors (esophageal stethoscope, pulse oximeter, end-tidal CO_2 monitors) are appropriate with assist devices. In addition to an arterial catheter, central venous and pulmonary artery catheters are useful for monitoring and for drug infusion. A left atrial line helps determine the functioning of the TAH.

CONCLUSION

Results appear to be quite encouraging in certain applications of mechanical support as a bridge to cardiac transplantation. No significant difference appears in the rate of subsequent transplantation with the type or design of pump used. However, a significant difference in the rate of ultimate hospital discharge is seen. Similar results are found with both electrical and pneumatic pumps used as univentricular assist devices. Centrifugal pumps appear equally efficacious but are limited by time.

Since the length of support is initially uncertain, their usefulness as bridging devices is questionable.

Registry results suggest poorer outcomes with TAH than with single or biventricular assist devices. Registry results indicate that univentricular support outcome is similar to that of orthotopic heart transplant that does not require circulatory support. Certainly, continued clinical trials will sort out which device is optimal in a given situation. Ideally, as devices and, perhaps more important, patient selection and management are improved, complications will be minimized and overall outcome will improve.

References

1. Copeland JG, Emergy RW, Levinson MM, Copeland J, McAleer MJ, Riley JE: The role of mechanical support and transplantation in treatment of patients with end-stage cardiomyopathy. Circulation (suppl II) 72:7, 1985
2. Miller CA, Pae WE Jr, Pierce WS: Combined Registry for the clinical use of mechanical ventricular assist devices: Postcardiotomy cardiogenic shock. ASAIO Trans 36:43, 1990
3. Kriett JM, Kaye MP: The Registry of the International Society for Heart Transplantation: Seventh official report, 1990. J Heart Transplant 9:323, 1990
4. Miller CA, Pae WE Jr, Pierce WS: Combined registry for the clinical use of mechanical ventricular assist pumps and the total artificial heart in conjunction with heart transplantation: Fourth official report, 1989. J Heart Transplant 4:453, 1990
5. High KM, Pierce WS, Skeehan TM: In Hensley FA, Martin DE, eds. The Practice of Cardiac Anesthesia, p. 650. Boston, Little Brown, 1990
6. Portner PM, Jassawalla JA, Chen H et al: A new dual pusher-plate left heart assist blood pump. Proceedings of the International Society of Artificial Organs, Artificial Organs, (suppl)3:361, 1979
7. Portner PM, Oyer PE, Jassawalla JS, et al: A totally implantable ventricular assist device for end-stage heart disease. In: Unger F, ed. Assisted circulation 2. Heidelberg: Springer-Verlag, 1984:122.
8. Reed CC, Stafford TB, eds. Cardiopulmonary Bypass, 2nd ed. Houston, Medical Press, p. 378, 1985
9. Nasu M, Okada Y, Fujiwara H et al: Transesophageal echocardiographic findings of intracardiac events during cardiac assist. Artif Organs 5:377, 1990
10. Kyo S, Matsumura M, Takamoto S, Omoto R: Transesophageal color Doppler echocardiography during mechanical assist circulation. ASAIO Trans 3:722, 1989
11. Deleuze PH, Liu Y, Tixier D et al: Centrifugal pump or pneumatic ventricle for short-term mechanical circulatory support? Int J Artif Organs 12:327, 1989

12. Bolman RM III, Cox JL, Marshall W et al: Circulatory support with a centrifugal pump as a bridge to cardiac transplantation. Ann Thorac Surg 47:108, 1989

13. Pennington DG, Merjavy JP, Swartz T et al: Clinical experience with a centrifugal pump ventricular assist device. ASAIO Trans 28:93, 1982

14. Kanter KR, McBride LR, Pennington DG et al: Bridging to cardiac transplantation with pulsatile ventricular assist devices. Ann Thorac Surg 46:134, 1988

15. Cabrol C, Solis E, Muneretto C et al: Orthotopic transplantation after implantation of a Jarvik 7 total artificial heart. J Thorac Cardiovasc Surg 97:342, 1989

16. Copeland JG, Smith RG, Icenogle TB, Rhenman B, Williams R, Vasu MA: Early experience with the total artifical heart as a bridge to cardiac transplantation. Surg Clin North Am 8:621, 1988

David R. Salter
Cornelius M. Dyke

Cardiopulmonary Dysfunction
5 | After Brain Death

A RATIONALE FOR CARDIAC DONOR MANAGEMENT

During the past decade, the number of cardiac transplant centers and transplant candidates has progressively increased while cardiac donor availability has remained constant. This relative scarcity of cardiac donors has dramatically influenced donor selection, and great efforts are being made to use as many of the hearts that are offered as possible. Hearts that may not have been considered for transplantation several years ago are now being accepted and transplanted successfully. Kormos and associates recently reviewed the influence of donor stability and ischemic time on subsequent recipient survival.[1] Their data suggested that assessment of traditional donor criteria over the telephone could be misleading, and with proper on-site evaluation and management many more donors might be made available. In their series, a number of patients on moderate inotropic support were discovered to be hypotensive because of hypovolemia rather than myocardial dysfunction. After appropriate volume replacement, they were weaned from inotropes and were considered to be suitable donors. The impetus to carefully preserve healthy hearts, as well as to resuscitate and salvage marginal hearts for transplantation, has kindled an exciting area of transplant research. The interaction between cardiac function, cerebral ischemia, and brain death is well recognized and has fascinated investigators for many years. Novitsky and coworkers have been prominent in examining this interplay and have applied their experimental findings clinically.[2–13] This chapter reviews some of the basic pathophysiologic changes that influence cardiopulmonary performance after brain death.

PATHOPHYSIOLOGY OF PULMONARY DYSFUNCTION

Pulmonary dysfunction after brain death may be a manifestation of pulmonary contusion after blunt injury, aspiration of blood or gastric contents, or over-enthusiastic volume resuscitation. Patients with severe head injuries may also develop neurogenic pulmonary edema.[14] Novitsky and colleagues reported pulmonary edema, diffuse hemorrhage, and capillary endothelial damage in 37% of brain-dead baboons. Brain death occurred within 20 minutes of tonsillar herniation, which was produced by rapid infusion of saline through a Foley catheter in the subdural space. Histologic evidence of myocardial injury—contraction bands, focal coagulative necrosis, myocytolysis, with edema formation and interstitial mononuclear cell infiltrate—was seen in 73% of animals. Extremely high left atrial pressures that transiently exceeded pulmonary artery pressures were observed in 9 of 11 animals (Fig. 5-1). An estimated 72% of total blood volume was shunted into the lungs. These data suggested a hydrostatic mechanism of disruption of pulmonary capillaries and pulmonary dysfunction.[9]

Moss and coworkers demonstrated that pretreatment of shock-model beagles with diphenylhydantoin almost entirely eliminated pulmonary hemorrhagic changes, focal atelectasis, and hyaline membranes that were universally present in the untreated animals. They postulated that pulmonary dysfunction occurred through hypothalamic mediation and increased pulmonary venular tone.[15] Its interesting that these changes were not observed in dogs with denervated lungs, further suggesting a cerebral etiology.[16,17] Other studies that used an isolated carotid perfusion system were able to reproduce pulmonary lesions in dogs that were undergoing hypoxemic perfusion.[18] Ironically, high levels of oxygen also provoked pulmonary injury that was not observed in anemic animals. The mechanism of injury was postulated to be inhibition of cerebral oxidative metabolism by high cellular oxygen levels. Brain lactate levels doubled, and cerebrospinal fluid potassium concentrations were elevated. Cerebrospinal fluid pseudocholinesterase rose tenfold.[19]

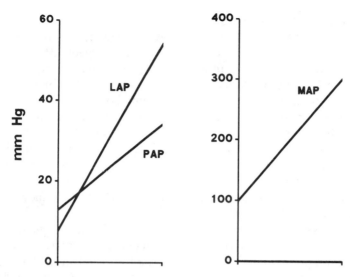

FIGURE 5-1. Mean changes in pulmonary arterial pressure, left atrial pressure, and systemic pressure from control levels to those at the peak of systemic vascular resistance during brain death in baboons. *PAP*, pulmonary arterial pressure (mm Hg); *LAP*, left atrial pressure (mm Hg); *MAP*, mean arterial pressure (mm Hg). *(Cooper DKC, Novitzky D (eds): Selection and management of the donor. In: The transplantation and replacement of thoracic organs, p. 44. Hingham, MA, Kluwer Academic Publishers, 1991)*

PATHOPHYSIOLOGY OF CARDIAC DYSFUNCTION

In the earliest series of donor hearts evaluated for transplantation at Stanford, none had a normal electrocardiogram (ECG).[20] The individual credited with first describing the relationship between cerebral injury and abnormalities of cardiopulmonary function was Cushing.[21] Novitsky and colleagues described five phases of ECG instability in the baboon.[2] Stage I was characterized by bradycardia followed by sinus arrest and complete heart block. In stage II, sinus tachycardia developed without ischemic changes. Multifocal ventricular ectopy was seen in stage III, and in stage IV sinus tachycardia (180 beats per minute) and ischemia were observed. Eventually (stage V), heart rates dropped to preinjury levels with a regular rhythm. These changes were observed over the course of several hours, and ECG abnormalities persisted in 50% of the animals studied.

Cardiac dysfunction has been observed not only in patients with brain death, but also in patients with severe head injuries and subarachnoid hemorrhage.[22,23] Of 23 patients examined 1 week after subarachnoid hemorrhage, a large subgroup who subsequently experienced a high morbidity and mortality rate were found to have a high incidence of elevated renin and urinary catecholamine levels.[24] Pollick and associates demonstrated echocardiographic wall motion abnormalities in 4 of 13 patients with subarachnoid hemorrhage.[25] The only deaths occurred in 3 of the 4 patients. Autopsy of 54 patients with subarachnoid hemorrhage revealed normal coronary arteries in 35 patients, small foci of inflammatory cells between the muscle fibers with or without the presence of necrotic muscle fibers in 30 patients, and hypothalamic and myocardial lesions in 42 patients.[26,27]

Because many patients with subarachnoid hemorrhage, as well as with brain death, have high circulating catecholamine levels, the concept of controlling systemic effects by the administration of β-blockers has intuitive appeal and appears to be effective in preventing myocardial necrosis.[28–36] Cruickshank and coworkers were the first to demonstrate a significant positive correlation between actual noradrenaline concentration and cardiac damage.[23] Myocardial injury has also been observed in rats after sudden increases in intracranial pressure.[37] Increases in intracranial pressure above diastolic pressure resulted in marked elevation of systemic pressure, which correlated directly with elevated catecholamines. The severity of ECG changes was prognostic of eventual fatal outcomes.

Novtizky and colleagues observed large decreases in free plasma triiodothyronine (T_3), thyroxine (T_4), plasma cortisol, and insulin levels after brain death in baboons.[2] Similarly, decreased T_3 levels have been found in human organ donors, and the extent of this reduction is related to the duration of the brain-dead state.[11] Further animal studies indicate a change from aerobic to anaerobic metabolism with rapid depletion of high-energy phosphates.[38] Administration of T_3 results in reversal of this metabolic derangement and substantial improvement of cardiac performance.[4]

PREOPERATIVE DONOR MANAGEMENT

The series of profound pathophysiologic events that occurs shortly after the onset of brain death makes management of these patients challenging. The time between cerebral injury and eventual organ donation is frequently lengthy, and it may be difficult for staff at the donor hospital to sustain an enthusiastic level of intensive care for a patient who has been declared brain dead. However, a successful outcome for the various organ recipients is critically dependent on meticulous management of each organ system during this pretransplantation phase.

Pulmonary Management

Brain death is accompanied by loss of brain stem function and dependence on mechanical ventilation. The goal of pulmonary care is to maintain oxygenation and prevent atelectasis and infection. Ventilation with tidal volumes of 10 to 15 mL/kg with positive end-expiratory pressure (PEEP) levels of 3 to 5 cm H_2O is applied. If the donor's lungs are to be used, it is desirable to avoid an inspired oxygen concentration (FiO_2) greater than 0.5 to limit the risk of oxygen toxicity. If injury precludes the use of the lungs as donor organs, a higher FiO_2 is preferable to high levels of PEEP to maintain Po_2 at 100 mm Hg because excessive PEEP may impair venous return and cardiac output and decrease perfusion of the liver and kidneys. Maintenance of adequate oxygenation is vital to the preservation of other organs for transplantation. If neurogenic pulmonary edema has occurred, use of higher levels of PEEP and fluid restriction may be necessary to achieve this goal. Hourly endotracheal suctioning and manual inflation are applied to prevent atelectasis and pneumonia.

Hemodynamic Management

The volume status of each donor must be precisely established. Criteria such as ideal weight, central venous pressure, pulmonary capillary wedge pressure, and recorded fluid balances are helpful. Patients who have sustained multiple injuries and who have endured multiple operative procedures may be hypervolemic and may require aggressive diuresis. Frequently, however, patients who have sustained lethal head injuries have been intentionally maintained in a relatively hypovolemic state to minimize cerebral swelling. Conventional resuscitation of the donor once an accurate volume status has been derived is to use lactated Ringer's solution for volume expansion. Volumes of 1 to 5 L may be required to restore the central venous pressure to 10 to 12 mm Hg. This initial volume load is followed by a maintenance infusion of 100 mL/h plus the previous hour's urine output. Patients are transfused as required to keep the hematocrit greater than 30%. Blood pressure should be maintained at greater than 90 mm Hg with central venous pressure within the normal range.

The cardiopulmonary consequences of brain death are considerable. As cerebral function progressively deteriorates and eventually results in brain death, a massive catecholamine surge occurs. Catecholamine levels in these patients are comparable only to those seen in cases of near-drowning, accidental catecholamine administration, and cocaine overdose. Adrenalin levels may be elevated as much as 11 times normal, noradrenaline levels tripled, and dopamine levels doubled.[2] This adrenergic storm results in microinfarcts in the heart, which can contribute to post-transplant heart failure.[7] Treatment should be initiated rapidly to minimize the adverse effects on the myocardium and lessen the likelihood of neurogenic pulmonary edema; it may be accomplished with the use of nitroprusside and short-acting β-blockers. An infusion of esmolol hydrochloride would seem to be ideal because its negative inotropic effects wane rapidly once the infusion is discontinued.[39]

Transient bradyarrhythmia (Cushing's reflex) may also be seen during the early hypertensive response to brain death. Treatment with atropine sulfate is ineffective; therefore, epinephrine or isoproterenol hydrochloride should be used if asystole or hypotension result. Supraventricular and ventricular arrhythmia may also occur as a result of the high levels of circulating catecholamines. If they do not respond to β-blocker therapy, short-term antiarrhythmic drugs may be administered.

The initial hypertensive crisis of brain death, regardless of its duration, is transient. Once destruction of the pontine and medullary vasomotor structures has occurred, the predominant hemodynamic abnormality is hypotension secondary to loss of arterial and venous vasomotor tone and volume depletion.[40] If volume expansion cannot be accomplished rapidly enough, or if it fails to result in reversal of the hypotension, an infusion of dopamine (2–10 μg/kg/min) may be added. Optimal function of the liver and kidney grafts does not occur if donor systolic pressure is allowed to remain below 80 mm Hg.[41,42] Therefore, it is recommended that systolic pressure be maintained in the range of 90 to 100 mm Hg. Isoproterenol and dobutamine are generally not helpful in this regard because of their vasodilatory effects. Excessive use of catecholamines should be avoided because of the increased oxygen consumption and decreased regional organ blood flow that may result.

The possibility of significant coronary artery disease must also be investigated. A history of hypertension or hyperlipidemia, particularly in the older donor, should raise suspicion. Not all donor institutions have the capability of angiographic evaluation of the donor heart, and therefore other methods should be considered. Wall motion abnormalities on echocardiogram, for example, may uncover the presence of an old infarct. In addition, ECG evidence of prior myocardial infarction may be found. Cooper and Novitzky have suggested the use of an isoproterenol stress test in which the heart rate is increased to 140 beats per minute and the ECG is carefully examined for evidence of ischemic changes.[43] Final confirmation of coronary artery disease is obtained while directly inspecting the heart and carefully palpating for evidence of atherosclerotic calcification or myocardial injury.

Thermal Regulation

Donors may also have difficulty with thermoregulation as a result of hypothalamic dysfunction. Core temperature should be monitored with a bladder, esophageal, or rectal temperature probe. Hypothermia may also result from the rapid infusion of unwarmed crystalloid or blood products. Active warming blankets, heating lamps, blood and fluid warmers, and humidified and heated inspired gases may be used to prevent or treat hypothermia. Body temperature should be maintained at greater than 35°C, several degrees above the fibrillation threshold. These patients can also become hyperthermic and require active cooling. Cultures should be drawn when this condition occurs, since sepsis may also be the cause.

Diabetes Insipidus

Destruction of the hypothalamic–pituitary axis that occurs from head trauma or global brain ischemia results in impaired secretion of antidiuretic hormone and central diabetes insipidus.[44] In the absence of antidiuretic hormone, water reabsorption is impaired in the cortical and medullary collecting tubules, resulting in the production of large amounts of dilute urine. This condition occurs in a majority of neurologically dead patients and may complicate fluid management by causing hypernatremia, hypokalemia, hypomagnesemia, or serious volume contraction.[45]

Aqueous vasopressin is administered in doses of 10 to 15 units every 2 to 4 hours, or as an infusion at a rate of 0.5 to 1.0 unit per hour. An infusion may be preferable to avoid the pressor response that is seen with intermittent intravenous doses. Augmentation of catecholamine therapy may also occur. Desmopressin acetate may be a preferred form of vasopressin therapy because of its longer duration of action and decreased pressor effect.[46]

The goal of vasopressin therapy is to keep urine output between 100 and 250 mL/h. Excessive administration of vasopressin should be avoided because it causes vasoconstriction, decreased splanchnic and renal perfusion, and, possibly, decreased cardiac output and pulmonary edema.[47,48]

Coagulopathy

Many donors exhibit some form of coagulopathy.[49] Clinically significant bleeding should be treated with component therapy to minimize intra-operative blood loss. Administration of ϵ-aminocaproic acid should be avoided because of the possibility of microvascular thrombosis.

Antibiotics

Although no data support their efficacy in preventing infectious compli-cations, some centers administer prophylactic antibiotics to the donor. Appropriate antibiotics should be administered when infection is sus-pected or confirmed.

Additional Therapy

The role of hormonal therapy in organ donors is still controversial. Nov-itzky and coworkers have demonstrated improvement in experimental animals and in human donors treated with cortisol, insulin, and T_3.[6,8,10] Brain death in pigs was accompanied by a reduction in myocardial energy stores that was associated with reduced myocardial function. Hormone therapy resulted in replenishment of myocardial energy and glycogen reserves, reduction in lactate, and improved cardiac function. Hormone-treated human donors, when compared with historic controls, exhibited improved cardiovascular status and required less inotropic support and bicarbonate. Organs from all treated donors were suitable for transplantation, whereas 20% of untreated donors were considered to be unsuitable as cardiac donors because of progressive cardiovascular deterioration or ventricular fibrillation.[11] Their current recommendation is the hourly administration of T_3 (2 μg), cortisol (100 mg), and insulin

(10–20 units) intravenously until blood-gas evidence shows that anaerobic metabolism has ceased.[50]

Although Macoviak and associates did not administer hormone therapy to 22 donors with low T_3 and T_4 levels, normal graft function was observed after cardiac transplantation.[51]

The role of oxygen-free radicals in reperfusion injury has prompted the proposed use of scavengers such as mannitol, steroids, deferoxamine, and superoxide dismutase to improve organ function.[52]

Monitoring and Laboratory

Central venous and arterial pressure lines are necessary to insure appropriate fluid and vasopressor therapy. Pulmonary artery catheters are rarely needed. Continuous temperature monitoring is essential. Arterial blood gases, serum electrolytes, hematocrit and hemoglobin levels, blood glucose and blood cultures, and chest x-rays are obtained as needed.

INTRAOPERATIVE MANAGEMENT OF THE CARDIAC DONOR

Continued meticulous care of the donor in the intraoperative phase of management is critical. Because these patients are frequently hemodynamically unstable and may be inotrope dependent, they must be transported with careful attention to moving infusion lines, arterial lines, and other "attachments." The coordinated transport of the donor requires a unique degree of cooperation between the anesthesiologist and various transplant surgeons. Prepping the patient for surgery should proceed precisely as a routine operative procedure, with the strictest attention to sterility.

Although the administration of anesthesia is unnecessary, muscle twitching due to spinal cord reflexes does occur and should be treated with muscle relaxants. Marked hypertension may occur with surgical stimulation and should be treated with vasodilating agents.

Vasoactive agents such as epinephrine, ephedrine, calcium, sodium nitroprusside, phenylephrine, and dopamine should be available to manage rapid changes in cardiovascular status. The position of the endotracheal tube should be checked after transfer to the operating table. Blood gases, electrolytes, and hematocrit and hemoglobin levels should be obtained at the beginning of the procedure and as necessary through-out. Adequate fluids (and a fluid warmer) should be available for volume replenishment. A warming blanket should be on the operating table. When multiple organs are to be procured by several teams, it is essential that the anesthesiologist communicate with each team and understand their particular needs.

DONOR CARDIECTOMY

The heart is exposed through a conventional median sternotomy incision that is extended to the symphysis if intra-abdominal organs are being harvested. Meticulous hemostasis is important to maintain a clean oper-ative field and minimize hemodynamic instability in an already precar-ious patient. Examination of the heart and mediastinum may reveal mediastinal hematomas or areas of bruising, which suggest either blunt trauma or an episode of external massage. Attempts at intracardiac injec-tion can also be detected. These suspicions are confirmed if blood is encountered within the pericardium. Since the heart will be opened, free floating debris in the pericardium, such as fat or bone wax, should be carefully retrieved to avoid inadvertent trapping within the heart and eventual embolization. Intravascular volume can be rapidly assessed by inspection of the right ventricular free wall and palpation of the pul-monary artery and outflow tract. This information is communicated to the anesthesiologist, who is then able to correlate this data with central venous pressure values and adjust therapy. It is not uncommon to open the pericardium in hypotensive, tachycardic patients and observe a small hypercontractile heart with low pulmonary artery pressures, a collapsing anterior right ventricular free wall, and pericardial fluid that has turned to foam. These findings suggest prolonged periods of unrecognized hypovolemia in a heart that has been stimulated by the massive release of endogenous catecholamines and the misguided administration of exogenous catecholamines. Rapid volume expansion readily corrects this situation and determines cardiac performance in a more physiologic vol-ume-loaded state. Clues from the preoperative history, ECG, and echo-cardiographic evaluation of the cardiac donor should be confirmed at this point. Signs of chronic hypertension may be present, with concentric left ventricular hypertrophy or atherosclerotic changes in the ascending aorta. The coronary arteries should be carefully palpated for evidence of disease and the myocardium inspected closely to detect areas of acute injury or areas of scarring. The accurate evaluation of right ventricular performance is critical for all recipients and especially for those with elevated pulmonary vascular resistance. Once the harvesting team has thoroughly evaluated the donor heart, a call to the recipient's hospital with a report and update of timing is always appreciated and, indeed, essential.

At this point, the cardiac surgical team is able to provide continuous feedback to the anesthesiologist and assist in coordinating the efforts of his or her harvesting colleagues from other specialties. Transesophageal echocardiography may be valuable to provide ongoing assessment of ventricular performance; however, it is not always readily available. Transesophageal visualization of the heart may also be difficult when the pericardium is suspended and the posterior aspect of the heart is no longer lying in contact with the posterior mediastinal tissues.

A standard routine for cardiac explantation is to secure a cardioplegia cannula to the ascending aorta and deliver 1 L of cold crystalloid antegrade cardioplegia after cross-clamping the aorta. For years, however, rapid extirpation and immediate immersion in ice slush was used— the Montezuma technique—with excellent results. Once the team is ready to excise the heart, 30,000 units of heparin are administered and the anesthesiologist is requested to withdraw the central lines so that they are not inadvertently cut when the superior vena cava is transected. The superior vena cava is then carefully ligated at least 1 cm above the atriocaval junction to avoid injury to the sinoatrial node and the need for a permanent pacemaker. The site of inferior caval transection is negotiated with the liver team. After transection, the heart is allowed to decompress itself for several beats. The aorta is then cross-clamped, and cardioplegia is delivered. At this point, the right superior pulmonary vein is transected and the left side of the heart is decompressed. Acute distention of the donor heart may result in added injury and increase the need for recipient inotropic support. Finally, the heart is excised by completing the transection of the pulmonary veins, pulmonary artery, aorta, and superior vena cava. Thorough inspection reveals any valvular abnormalities, atrial septal defect, patent foramen ovale, or other anomalies. The heart is then carefully washed and placed in iced saline in three plastic bags with all air evacuated and transported on ice. It is important not to allow the heart to lie in direct contact with the ice, since this contact may create regional hypothermic injuries.

Presently, further management of the donor heart during its transition between owners is suspended. Future advances will likely focus on using this transitional period to begin actively resuscitating the myocardium with myocardial metabolic additives or modulating the deleterious effects of free radicals.

CONCLUSION

Recent advances in understanding the pathophysiology of brain death have greatly enhanced the ability of intensivists, surgeons, and anesthesiologists to manage organ donors. Continued research efforts to examine these fascinating clinical problems of donor management hold great promise for future insights into numerous mysteries, such as hormonal regulation of the heart.

References

1. Kormos RL, Donato W, Hardesty RL et al: The influence of donor organ stability and ischemia time on subsequent cardiac recipient survival. Transpl Proc 20:980, 1988
2. Novitzky D, Wicomb WN, Cooper DKC et al: Electrocardiographic, haemodynamic and endocrine changes occurring during experimental brain death in the Chacma baboon. J Heart Transplant 4:63, 1984
3. Novitzky D, Cooper DKC, Wicomb WN et al: Brain death-induced hemodynamic changes resulting in cardiac and pulmonary injury in the baboon. Transplant Proc 18:1190, 1986
4. Novitzky D, Wicomb WN, Cooper DKC et al: Evidence of myocardial and renal functional recovery following hormonal treatment after brain death. Transplant Proc 18:613, 1986
5. Wicomb WN, Cooper DKC, Lanza RP et al: The effects of brain death and 24 hours' storage by hypothermic perfusion on donor heart function in the pig. J Thorac Cardiovasc Surg 91:896, 1986
6. Novitzky D, Wicomb WN, Cooper DKC et al: Improved function of stored hearts following hormonal therapy after brain death in pigs. Transplant Proc 18:1419, 1986
7. Novitzky D, Wicomb WN, Cooper DKC et al: Prevention of myocardial injury during brain death by total cardiac sympathectomy in the Chacma baboon. Ann Thorac Surg 41:520, 1986
8. Novitzky D, Wicomb WN, Cooper DKC et al: Improved cardiac function following hormonal therapy in brain dead pigs: Relevance to organ donation. Cryobiology 24:1, 1987
9. Novitzky D, Wicomb WN, Rose AG et al: Pathophysiology of pulmonary edema following experimental brain death in the Chacma baboon. Ann Thorac Surg 43:288, 1987
10. Novitzky D, Cooper DKC, Reichart B: The value of hormonal therapy in improving organ viability in the transplant donor. Transplant Proc 19:2037, 1987
11. Novitzky D, Cooper DKC, Reichart B: Hemodynamic and metabolic responses to hormonal therapy in brain-dead potential organ donors. Transplantation 43:852, 1987
12. Novitzky D, Human PA, Cooper DKC: Inotropic effect of triiodothyronine following myocardial ischemia and cardiopulmonary bypass: An experimental study in pigs. Ann Thorac Surg 45:50, 1988

13. Novitzky D, Rose AG, Cooper DKC: Injury of myocardial conduction tissue and coronary artery smooth muscle following brain death in the baboon. Transplantation 45:964, 1988
14. Ducker TB: Increased intracranial pressure and pulmonary edema. I. Clinical study of 11 patients. J Neurosurg 28:112, 1968
15. Stein AA, Moss G: Cerebral etiology of the respiratory distress syndrome: Diphenylhydantoin (DPH) prophylaxis. Surgical Forum 24:433, 1973
16. Dworkin P, Moss G: Cerebral etiology of the pulmonary lesions of "oxygen toxicity." Surgical Forum 24:211, 1973
17. Moss G, Stein AA: The centrineurogenic etiology of the respiratory distress syndrome. (Induction by isolated cerebral hypoxemia and prevention by unilateral pulmonary denervation.) Am J Surg 132:352, 1976
18. Moss G, Staunton C, Stein AA: Cerebral etiology of the "shock lung syndrome." J Trauma 12:885, 1972
19. Moss G, Stein AA: Cerebral etiology of the acute respiratory distress syndrome: Diphenylhydantoin prophylaxis. J Trauma 15:39, 1975
20. Griepp RB, Stinson EB, Clark DA et al: The cardiac donor. Surg Gynecol Obstet 132:792, 1971
21. Cushing H: Concerning a definite regulatory mechanism of the vasomotor center which controls blood pressure during cerebral compression. Johns Hopkins Hospital Bulletin 12:290, 1901
22. McLeod AA, Neil-Dwyer G, Meyer CHA et al: Cardiac sequelae of acute head injury. Br Heart J 47:221, 1982
23. Cruickshank JM, Neil-Dwyer G, Stott AW: Possible role of catecholamines, corticosteroids, and potassium in production of electrocardiographic abnormalities associated with subarachnoid hemorrhage. Br Heart J 36:697, 1974
24. Neil-Dwyer G, Walter P, Shaw HJH et al: Plasma renin activity in patients after a subarachnoid hemorrhage: A possible predictor of outcome. Neurosurgery 7:578, 1980
25. Pollick C, Cujec B, Parker S et al: Left ventricular wall motion abnormalities in subarachnoid hemorrhage: An echocardiographic study. J Am Coll Cardiol 12:600, 1988
26. Doshi R, Neil-Dwyer GN: Hypothalamic and myocardial lesions after subarachnoid hemorrhage. J Neurol Neurosurg Psychiatry 40:821, 1977
27. Doshi R, Neil-Dwyer G: A clinicopathological study of patients following a subarachnoid hemorrhage. J Neurosurg 52:295, 1980
28. Neil-Dwyer G, Walter P, Cruickshank JM: Beta-blockade benefits patients following a subarachnoid haemorrhage. Eur J Clin Pharmacol [suppl]28:25, 1985
29. Cruickshank JM, Neil-Dwyer G: Beta-blocker brain concentrations in man. Eur J Clin Pharmacol [suppl]28:25, 1985
30. Neil-Dwyer G, Cruickshank JM: Plasma renin and angiotensin II levels in subarachnoid hemorrhage. J Neurol Sci 23:463, 1974
31. Neil-Dwyer G, Mee E, Dorrance D et al: Early intervention with nimodipine in subarachnoid hemorrhage. Eur Heart J 8:41, 1987
32. Mee E, Dorrance D, Lowe D et al: Controlled study of nimodipine in aneurysm patients treated early after subarachnoid hemorrhage. Neurosurgery 22:484, 1988
33. Neil-Dwyer G, Cruickshank J, Stratton C: Beta-blockers, plasma total creatine kinase and creatine kinase myocardial isoenzyme and the prognosis of subarachnoid hemorrhage. Surg Neurol 25:163, 1986

34. Cruickshank JM, Neil-Dwyer G, Cameron MM et al: Beta-adrenoceptor-blocking agents and the blood-brain barrier. Clin Sci 59:453S, 1980
35. Neil-Dwyer G, Walter P, Cruickshank JM et al: Effect of propanolol and phentolamine on myocardial necrosis after subarachnoid hemorrhage. Br Med J 2:990, 1978
36. Neil-Dwyer G, Cruickshank J, Stott A et al: The urinary catecholamine and plasma cortisol levels in patients with subarachnoid hemorrhage. J Neurol Sci 22:375, 1974
37. Shanlin RJ, Sole MJ, Rahimifar M et al: Changes in plasma catecholamine levels after insula damage in experimental stroke. Brain Res 375:182, 1986
38. Novitzky D, Cooper DKC, Morrell D, Isaacs S: Change from aerobic to anaerobic metabolism after brain death and reversal following triiodothyronine (T_3) therapy. Transplantation 45:32, 1988
39. Darby JM, Stein KS, Grenvik A, Stuart SA: Approach to management of the heartbeating 'brain dead' organ donor. JAMA 261:2222, 1989
40. Emery RW, Cork RC, Levinson MM et al: The cardiac donor: A six-year experience. Ann Thorac Surg 41:356, 1986
41. Whelchel JD, Diethelm AG, Philips MG, Rhyder Wr, Schein LG: The effect of high-dose dopamine in cadaver donor management on delayed graft function and graft survival following renal transplantation. Transplant Proc 18:523, 1986
42. Busuttil RW, Goldstein Li, Danovitch GM, Ament ME: Liver transplantation today. Ann Intern Med 104:377, 1986
43. Cooper DKC, Novitzky D (eds.): Selection and management of the donor. In The Transplantation and Replacement of Thoracic Organs, p. 41. Hingham, MA, Kluwer Academic Publishers, 1991.
44. Outwater KM, Rockoff MA: Diabetes insipidus accompanying brain death in children. Neurology 34:1243, 1984
45. Copeland JG, Emery RW, Levinson MM et al: Selection of patients for cardiac transplantation. Circulation 75:2, 1987
46. Richardson DW, Robinson AG: Desmopressin. Ann Intern Med 103:228, 1985
47. Richardson PDI, Witherington PG: Liver blood flow. II. Effects of drugs on hormones in liver blood flow. Gastroenterology 81:356, 1981
48. Schneider A, Toledo-Pereyra LH, Zeichner WD et al: Effect of dopamine and pitressin on kidneys procured and harvested for transplantation. Transplantation 36:110, 1982
49. Kaufman HH, Hui KS, Mattson JC et al: Clinicopathologic correlations of disseminated intravascular coagulation in patients with severe head injury. Neurosurgery 15:34, 1984
50. Novitzky D, Cooper DKC, Human P, et al: Triiodothyronine therapy for heart donor and recipient. J Heart Transplant 7:370, 1988
51. Macoviak JA, McDougall IR, Bayer MF et al: Significance of thyroid dysfunction in human cardiac allograft procurement. Transplantation 43:824, 1987
52. Stewart JR, Berhardt EB, Wehr CJ et al: Free radical scavengers and myocardial preservation during transplantation. Ann Thorac Surg 42:390, 1986

J. Olak
G. A. Patterson

6 Single-Lung Transplantation, 1991

The modern era of human single-lung transplantation began at the University of Toronto in 1983 under the direction of Dr. J. D. Cooper, representing the culmination of about 40 years of clinical and laboratory investigation on the subject.

In 1947, the Russian physiologist Demikhov homografted canine pulmonary lobes.[1] Shortly thereafter, both Metras in France and Juvenelle in the United States published their techniques of canine lung allo-transplantation.[2,3] On June 11, 1963, Hardy performed the first successful human single-lung transplantation. His patient, a 58-year-old male with a carcinoma of the left main bronchus, emphysema, and chronic renal insufficiency, died on the 18th postoperative day of renal failure and malnutrition.[4] Over the next 6 years, 20 surgeons attempted a total of 22 lung transplants with only one long-term survivor.[5] Derom's single-lung transplant in a patient with silicosis functioned for 10 months. Of interest is the fact that this graft was neither cooled, ventilated, nor perfused during its 50-minute ischemic time.[6]

Poor early results have been attributed to a variety of factors, including poor donor-organ selection, poor recipient selection, inadequate organ preservation, suboptimal immunosuppression, infection, and technical problems that involved the bronchial anastomosis. Research at the University of Toronto and elsewhere addressed many of these issues between 1968 and 1983.

St. LOUIS LUNG TRANSPLANT REGISTERY
SINGLE LUNG TRANSPLANTS PER YEAR

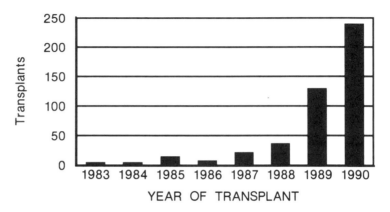

FIGURE 6-1. Growth in the number of single-lung transplants by year worldwide. *(Courtesy of the St. Louis Lung Transplant Registry, February 1991)*

The introduction of cyclosporine immunosuppression in the early 1980s revolutionized solid organ transplantation. Lung transplantation is now considered to be a viable treatment option for selected patients with end-stage lung disease. The operative technique is rapidly becoming standardized and lung transplantation can no longer be considered experimental.

Currently, both the International Society for Heart Transplantation and Washington University in St. Louis maintain lung transplantation registries. Their data indicate that the annual number of single-lung transplants exceeded 100 per year worldwide for the first time in 1989 (Fig. 6-1). By February 28, 1991, Washington University had registered a total of 415 single-lung transplants in 395 recipients. The actuarial 1-year survival is 64%. Established programs, such as those at the University of Toronto, Washington University, Stanford University, and the University of Texas at San Antonio, report actuarial 2-year survival near 60%. This percentage is expected to increase as the number of early deaths declines.[7]

As of February 28, 1991, 63 lung transplant centers, 52 of which were American, had submitted cases to the Washington University Lung Transplant Registry. The majority of centers had performed less than five transplants in the previous 12-month period.

INDICATIONS AND SELECTION OF RECIPIENTS

Initially, only patients with idiopathic pulmonary fibrosis, hypersensitivity pneumonitis, or other fibrotic lung diseases were considered for single-lung transplantation at the University of Toronto. Beginning in 1988, however, selected patients with nonbullous emphysema were accepted into the program. The indications for single-lung transplantation were further broadened that same year to include selected patients with primary pulmonary hypertension and pulmonary hypertension secondary to Eisenmenger's physiology. Registry data indicate that about two thirds of the single-lung transplants performed to date have been for either pulmonary fibrosis or emphysema (Fig. 6-2).

Current selection criteria include the following:

1. Age less than 60 years
2. Absence of major systemic illness or end-organ failure
3. No previous major thoracic surgery
4. No or minimal systemic steroids (5 mg prednisone/day)
5. Ambulatory with rehabilitation potential
6. Adequate nutritional status; within 10% of ideal body weight

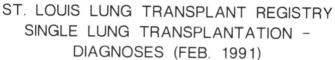

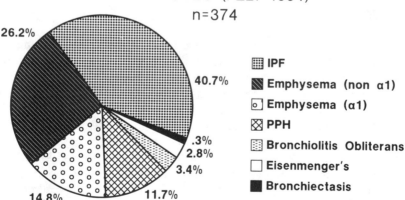

FIGURE 6-2. Diagnoses of single-lung transplant recipients. *IPF*, idiopathic pulmonary fibrosis; *PPH*, primary pulmonary hypertension. *(Courtesy of the St. Louis Lung Transplant Registry, February 1991)*

7. No major psychiatric or substance-abuse history
8. Psychosocial and financial support

It has always been considered important to offer transplantation to patients in whom all other therapeutic options have been exhausted and in whom life expectancy is predicted to be between 6 and 18 months without transplantation.

Criteria have been modified as experience has been gained. Systemic steroid use, for example, is no longer considered an absolute contraindication to single-lung transplantation. Recent research indicates that its use may not be as detrimental to bronchial anastomotic healing as was once thought.[8] Right heart function criteria have been relaxed as well, with the realization that techniques available for the assessment of recoverability of right heart function are not yet sufficiently accurate.

In Toronto, a total of 645 referrals for possible lung transplantation were received between 1983 and April 1990. Forty-five percent of referred patients were refused after initial screening. The most common reasons were advanced age, steroid use, multisystem disease, general debility, or psychosocial problems. Thirty percent underwent formal in-hospital evaluation. Ten percent of patients died while waiting for assessment, and 3% died while on the active waiting list. Only 10% of patients referred to the program were transplanted, while 2% are on an active waiting list.

DONOR MANAGEMENT AND SELECTION

The rate-limiting step in lung transplantation has been the shortage of suitable donor organs. The Canadian organ procurement agency, Multiorgan Retrieval and Exchange, has estimated that, of all patients offered as organ donors, only 5% to 10% have lungs suitable for harvesting, in contrast to 24% for livers and 94% for kidneys.

Many reasons for this shortage can be found. The majority of lung donors suffer brain death as a result of intracerebral hemorrhage or trauma. Aspiration commonly complicates these events, precluding lung donation. In addition, head-injured patients often develop diabetes insipidus, which increases the potential for developing pulmonary edema, thereby jeopardizing an otherwise suitable lung graft. Other injuries associated with trauma may necessitate initial administration of massive amounts of fluid and likewise contribute to the development of pulmonary edema.

The situation is complex, since most patients have the potential to donate multiple organs; and each organ, in turn, has an optimal prehar-vest management plan that may be at variance with that of the others. For example, the renal team would rather the kidney donor have an expanded intravascular volume to insure adequate perfusion of the kidney; however, this volume might compromise pulmonary graft function by rendering it edematous. Suggested guidelines for the management of multiple organ donors include the following:[9]

1. Maintain mean arterial blood pressure above 70 mm Hg
2. Maintain central venous pressure below 10 mm Hg; pulmonary capillary wedge pressure below 12 mm Hg
3. Maintain blood pressure with vasopressors, preferably, instead of volume: dopamine 2.5 to 10 μ/kg/min; phenylephrine 0.06 to 0.18 mg/min
4. Treat diabetes insipidus:
    Administer vasopressin 5 to 10 Units every 8 hours or desmopressin acetate 0.3 μg/kg intravenously (IV) over 30 minutes
    Run IV fluids at 100 mL/hr plus the previous hour's urine output to maintain urine output at 1 mL/kg/h
    Replace electrolyte losses
5. Maintain normothermia
6. Maintain PaO_2 above 100 mm Hg on the lowest FIO_2 possible
7. Maintain positive end-expiratory pressure (PEEP) at 5 cm H_2O
8. Maintain strict pulmonary toilet; suction every 2 hours with $\pm$ NaCl instillation
9. Monitor arterial blood gases every 2 hours
10. Elevate head of bed if possible

Because pulmonary grafts are in short supply and their prolonged preservation has been more problematic than other organs, efforts to maximize their numbers should be made a priority in all critical care units. This effort demands vigorous care of the brain-dead patient in the hours preceding organ harvest.

Of prime importance is the use of vasopressors to maintain blood pressure when the intravascular space is replete. This has not been found to be detrimental to cardiac, renal, or hepatic graft function and helps to optimize pulmonary graft function.

Maintenance of the PaO_2 level above 100 mm Hg on the lowest FIO_2 possible with PEEP of 5 cm H_2O is accomplished by suctioning the airway as often as necessary and by using bronchodilators as required. Arterial blood gases should be monitored every 2 hours, and supine chest x-rays should be repeated every 4 hours so that necessary adjustments to ventilator settings can be made.

The optimal lung donor is a patient younger than 55 years of age who is a life-long nonsmoker free of pulmonary disease or thoracic trauma. In addition to being ABO compatible and HIV- and hepatitis-negative, the prospective donor must be a good size match. He or she must also be hemodynamically stable and have clear serial portable chest radiographs, a PaO_2 above 300 mm Hg on 100% oxygen and 5 cm PEEP, a negative gram stain of the tracheal aspirate, and a bronchoscopy exam that fails to reveal grossly purulent secretions or evidence of aspiration. Immediately before lung harvest, a manual and visual inspection is undertaken to insure that no contusions or significant pleural adhesions are present. Some centers also require a cytomegalovirus (CMV) serology match, hoping that this match will decrease reactivation and pneumonitis in the post-transplant period.

PRESERVATION

A safe ischemic time for human pulmonary grafts is currently considered to be 4 to 6 hours.[10-13] This time limitation mandates close communication between procurement and recipient teams throughout the period leading up to the return of the pulmonary graft to the recipient hospital. In general, this constraint limits flying time between donor and recipient hospitals to about 2 hours.

While simple immersion, pulmonary flush, and core cooling have all been used to preserve lungs in the past, either of the latter two methods in combination with the first is more commonly used today. Most centers pretreat the donor with prostaglandin E_1 (500 μg) and then use a cold (4°C) prostaglandin E_1 modified EuroCollin's pulmonary flush (60 mL/ kg) to accomplish metabolic inhibition. The graft is immersed in cold (4°C) EuroCollin's solution for transport.

Research indicates that the period of safe ischemia for human pulmonary grafts may be lengthened by steroid or hormonal manipulation of the donor,[14,15] by further modification of the flush,[16,17] or by further modifications of operative and anesthetic techniques. The administration of oxygen free-radical scavengers at reflow in the in vitro canine lobar ischemic model attenuates reperfusion injury as evidenced by decreases in extracellular lung water after long-term (24-hour) hypothermic preservation.[15] This finding has not translated into a benefit in human lung transplantation.

When administered during the ischemic period, verapamil, a calcium channel blocker and vasodilator, significantly reduces tissue damage after 3 hours (range 2–5 hours) of normothermic ischemia, as evidenced by increased O_2 tension and decreased pulmonary vascular resistance in the in situ ischemic canine lung injury model.[18] It is not certain whether this reduction is due to its calcium channel blocking effect or its vasodilatory effect. Verapamil has also been shown to improve preservation when administered before extraction in the hypothermic, isolated, ventilated rabbit lung perfusion model. Its effect appears to be enhanced when used with extracellular flush solutions, such as low potassium dextran, and extended periods of preservation (48 hours).[19]

Current research that is focusing on alterations in endothelial cell membrane receptors using monoclonal antibody may result in prolongation of the period of safe ischemia by attenuating ischemia–reperfusion injury.

Improvement in the ability to preserve pulmonary grafts will enable coast-to-coast travel and maximize the potential for use of every suitable donor organ.

LUNG HARVEST

During lung harvest, the donor's intravascular volume and ventilatory status need to be continuously evaluated by the anesthesiologist to insure maintenance of a central venous pressure below 10 mm Hg and an adequate PaO_2. As in the preharvest phase, this period demands constant vigilance to avoid any deterioration of graft function before extraction. Dopamine, phenylephrine, blood, and blood products should be available in the operating room at all times. Arterial blood gas determinations should be made at 30-minute intervals on an F_{IO_2} of 1.0 and PEEP 5 cm H_2O to enable necessary adjustments in ventilation to be made. Care should also be taken to keep the donor's airway free of secretions and mucous plugs.

Once the liver and kidney and pancreas teams have mobilized their grafts, the cardiac team prepares the heart for extraction by placing a cardioplegic tack in the aortic root. The pulmonary team then places an 18F perfusion cannula midway between the pulmonary valve and the pulmonary artery bifurcation and, after alerting the other harvesting teams, injects 1000 μg of prostaglandin E_1 directly into the main pulmonary artery. The aorta is simultaneously cross-clamped and all organs are flushed. Throughout this phase, the lungs remain ventilated with tidal volumes of at least 20 mL/kg to insure uniform distribution of the pulmonary flush. Donor cardiectomy is then performed, followed by en bloc removal of the lungs using a technique described by the Toronto Lung Transplant Group.[20] Ventilation should be continued until the trachea has been stapled to minimize atelectasis. Immediately before tracheal stapling, the anesthesiologist is asked to manually ventilate the donor and to maintain a continuous airway pressure of 30 cm H_2O to enable immersion of the fully inflated lung bloc in cold EuroCollin's solution. The triple-bagged lung bloc is then packed in an ice chest for transport.

ANESTHETIC TECHNIQUE FOR SINGLE-LUNG TRANSPLANTATION

Anesthesia for lung transplantation demands modifications in existing techniques and tailoring of the approach to suit the recipient's underlying lung disease. This effort requires careful consideration of the pathophysiologic changes that accompany the patient's lung disease. Preoperative assessment of potential lung transplant recipients involves an evaluation of cardiac, pulmonary, and renal function. The results of pulmonary function and exercise testing using a modified Bruce protocol, ventilation/perfusion and radionuclide angiographic scanning, two-dimensional echocardiography, and, in selected cases, coronary angiography and right heart catheterization, are all reviewed. The primary anesthetic related consideration in the preoperative assessment of a potential lung transplant recipient is whether or not cardiopulmonary bypass is likely to be required. It has been observed that the preoperative room air PaO_2 (39 vs. 56.3 mm Hg), mean pulmonary artery pressure (45.3 vs. 30.9 mm Hg), and pulmonary vascular resistance (546.3 vs. 261.5 dyne/cm^2) of 3 Toronto patients who required bypass was significantly different ($P < 0.001$) from 12 who did not.[21] These and other parameters may be reliable predictors of the need for cardiopulmonary bypass.

Intraoperative monitoring includes electrocardiography, arterial line, pulmonary artery catheter, cardiac output, pulse oximetry, end-tidal CO_2, and temperature. A warming blanket is placed under the patient, and intravenous fluid warmers are used. The cardiopulmonary bypass machine is primed as soon as the procurement team reports that they will be harvesting. Both pediatric and adult bronchoscopes are on hand, the former to assess the bronchial anastomosis while the double lumen endotracheal tube is still in place, and the later to aspirate airway secretions after changing to a single lumen endotracheal tube at the conclusion of the transplant.

Induction of anesthesia is deliberately slow and controlled, with all drugs carefully titrated to the individual's response. Induction is typically accomplished with fentanyl citrate or sufentanil and incremental doses (25 mg) of thiopental sodium. Isoflurane or halothane have also been used with favorable results; the latter is preferred when a need for bronchodilatation is anticipated. The patient is paralyzed with either succinylcholine chloride, pancuronium bromide, or vecuronium. Both ketamine and etomidate have been used with success, the former being favored in patients with reactive airways.

For right lung transplants, a left-sided double lumen tube is used, whereas for left lung transplants a single lumen endotracheal tube and a bronchoscopically placed left-sided bronchial blocker (#14 F Fogarty embolectomy catheter) may be used. More recently, the Washington University group has described use of a left-sided double lumen endotracheal tube for all cases.

Ventilation is instituted using volumes of 8 to 10 mL/kg at a rate of 12 to 20 breaths per minute and an FiO_2 sufficient to maintain an oxygen saturation of 100%.

If tolerated by the patient, recipient pneumonectomy is performed with the lung collapsed. The final determination of the need for cardiopulmonary bypass is made during this phase of the operation. The recipient pulmonary artery is clamped, with the patient receiving 100% oxygen. The right atrium and right ventricle are observed for the development of dilatation and failure. If the patient becomes unstable, pharmacologic manipulation is attempted. Prostaglandin E_1, dobutamine, isoproterenol, and amrinone have all been used in selected circumstances. If, despite these measures, the arterial O_2 saturation remains below 90% on an FiO_2 of 1, the mixed venous O_2 remains less than 60%, or the cardiac index remains below 2.0 $L/min/m^2$, cardiopulmonary bypass is instituted. Femorofemoral bypass may be used for left lung transplants and aorta-to-right-atrial bypass for right lung transplants. Flow rates for patients who require cardiopulmonary bypass average 2.5 to 3.0 L/min.

SURGICAL TECHNIQUE FOR SINGLE-LUNG TRANSPLANTATION

Ideally, the side chosen for transplantation should depend on the results of preoperative differential lung function tests. Other factors, such as previous thoracic surgery, the presence of bullous disease in patients with emphysema, the status of the donor lungs, and the likelihood of having to use cardiopulmonary bypass, may also enter into the decision. Some groups prefer to transplant the right side in patients with emphysema because they feel that the left hemidiaphragm descends more readily to accommodate the hyperinflated native left lung, thereby pre-venting too much mediastinal shift toward the transplanted side.

From a technical point of view, the side chosen makes little differ-ence. It is preferable to transplant the right side when cardiopulmonary bypass is anticipated because aorto–atrial cannulation is more easily accomplished.

Because ischemic time remains a critical issue in lung transplanta-tion, the potential recipient is brought into the operating room and pre-pared for surgery while the donor operation is being performed. Only after the procurement team has fully assessed the potential lung graft and found it to be satisfactory is the recipient anesthetized. A standard posterolateral thoracotomy incision is used. The aim is to have the recip-ient vessels and bronchus completely dissected by the time the graft arrives in the operating room to further minimize ischemic time. Recip-ient pneumonectomy is completed when the graft is either close by or in the operating room. Timing is more critical for the bilateral sequential single-lung operation and with the more remote harvest. Many centers prepare the femoral vessels for possible cannulation and mobilize an omental pedicle through a short upper midline abdominal incision dur-ing the early phase of the operation. Once mobilized, the omentum is tucked into a retrosternal tunnel and used subsequently to wrap the bronchial anastomosis to control small dehiscences and to separate the bronchial suture line from the pulmonary arterial anastomosis. The bronchial anastomosis is completed first. The membranous wall is sewn first, then the cartilaginous portion is approximated, telescoping the donor bronchus into the recipient bronchus for a length of one car-tilaginous ring.

Because the lung is the only solid organ that is consistently trans-planted without re-establishing a systemic arterial connection, it used to be felt that an unacceptable rate of bronchial anastomotic problems would result from the perioperative use of steroids.[22] Although the only indication for steroid use in the early postoperative period had been the treatment of acute rejection, recent studies have demonstrated reliable bronchial healing despite their administration.[8,23]

Both Pinsker and associates and Cooper and colleagues have dem-onstrated that the incidence of bronchial complications is directly related to the length of the donor bronchus.[24,25] They noted that the anastomoses narrowed by 25% after reimplantation, indicating an ischemic etiology. Therefore, the donor bronchus is trimmed to within one to two cartilag-inous rings of the upper lobe bronchus takeoff. In an elegant series of canine experiments, Cooper and colleagues demonstrated that an autotransplanted ischemic left main bronchial stump could be revascularized by an omental wrap.[25] Bronchial omentopexy thus became part of the original surgical technique. The incidence of bronchial anastomotic complications has declined dramatically with the adaptation of a technique first described in dogs in the 1950s by Veith and recently repopularized in humans by Trinkle. It involves telescoping the donor bronchus into the recipient bronchus for a distance of at least one cartilaginous ring.[26] Both dehiscence and stricture rates appear to be markedly diminished with these technical changes. Results have improved so much that some surgeons no longer find it necessary to use an omental wrap. However, it is still advisable to use the omental wrap for cases when technical difficulties preclude performance of a perfect anastomosis.

After completion of the bronchial anastomosis, the pulmonary arterial anastomosis is completed, followed by the left atrial anastomosis. Antegrade de-airing is accomplished immediately before completion of the left atrial anastomosis by releasing the pulmonary arterial clamp. Immediately before de-airing, the graft is gently inflated to assess for air leak and to re-expand atelectatic areas, thereby avoiding shunt and decreasing pulmonary vascular resistance. Next, a pediatric bronchoscope is used to inspect the anastomosis for both patency and viability. If omentum is used, it may be wrapped around the bronchial anastomosis at this juncture. Two chest tubes are placed to evacuate air and fluid from the pleural space, and the chest is closed in standard fashion. The endotracheal tube is exchanged for a single lumen tube, and the tracheobronchial tree is cleared of secretions with an adult bronchoscope because of its larger suction channel. The patient is then transferred to the intensive care unit. A thoracic epidural catheter is placed within 12 hours of surgery, if possible, and is left in position for up to 5 days for the administration of postoperative analgesia.

POST-TRANSPLANTATION CARE AND SURVEILLANCE

Once in the intensive care unit, the patient is kept ventilated and sedated until hemodynamically stable. As soon as possible thereafter, the patient is weaned from the ventilator and extubated. This process usually occurs within 24 to 72 hours of surgery. Although early extubation is advantageous in most cases, patients with primary pulmonary hypertension who undergo single-lung transplantation frequently require 5 to 7 days of postoperative ventilation to enable their heart and lungs to adapt. In this group of patients, blood flows preferentially to the transplanted lung from the outset because of its more compliant vascular bed. This fact puts the new lung at risk for the development of reperfusion pulmonary injury, which can increase ventilation–perfusion mismatch. Any stimulus that increases cardiac output (e.g., agitation, pain, movement) may further increase the shunt and result in desaturation.

The safest approach for ventilating patients with emphysema is to use small tidal volumes and no PEEP. This approach helps to avoid development of air trapping in the native lung and subsequent mediastinal shift toward the transplanted side. For this reason, bilateral bullous disease is considered to be a contraindication to single-lung transplantation. Hyperinflation of the native lung has, on occasion, produced the need for surgery to reduce compression of the transplanted side and enable successful weaning from mechanical ventilation.

Intravenous (IV) fluids should be administered cautiously in the postoperative period to avoid both pulmonary edema and oliguria. Enteral nutrition using the nasoduodenal route is often started in the early postoperative period, reflecting the borderline nutritional status of many patients with end-stage lung disease. Parenteral alimentation is reserved for selected patients with postoperative ileus (e.g., those in whom the omentum was mobilized). Chest physiotherapy is started immediately. Patients are mobilized within the first 24 hours (except those who require heavy sedation). In Toronto, it has been observed that patients with chronic respiratory failure are more readily weaned from mechanical ventilation after they have been fully mobilized.

Immunosuppressive regimens vary between institutions, but most use an approach that includes cyclosporine, azathioprine, and steroid. Induction is sometimes accomplished with antilymphocyte globulin, which is continued until cyclosporine levels stabilize (usually 4–7 days). Until recently, steroids were avoided for the first 2 to 3 weeks after transplantation because of canine evidence that demonstrated poor bronchial anastomotic healing.[23] In Toronto, methylprednisolone (500 mg IV) is now given intraoperatively followed by methylprednisolone (2 mg/kg IV) for 5 days. Oral steroid (prednisone 0.5 mg/kg/day) is started thereafter and is tapered to 15 mg every other day by 12 months.

Cyclosporine is currently administered by continuous infusion in the early postoperative period to establish whole blood radioimmune assay levels between 250 and 340 ng/mL. Oral cyclosporine is started on a twice daily schedule with the return of gastrointestinal tract function. Cyclosporine levels are monitored daily until discharge from the hospital and weekly thereafter.

Azathioprine (1 mg/kg) is administered once daily. The dose is adjusted as necessary to maintain the white blood cell count above $4000/mm^3$ and the total lymphocyte count above $1000/mm^3$.

Some centers have included monoclonal antilymphocyte antibody (OKT3) in their immunosupression regimen, both as prophylaxis against rejection and for rejection refractory to bolus steroid therapy.[27]

In Toronto, antibiotic prophylaxis generally takes the form of a third generation cephalosporin, with or without clindamycin, until the perioperative donor and recipient sputum culture results are available. If the cultures are negative, antibiotics are discontinued; if they are positive, the patient is given a therapeutic course of an appropriate antibiotic. Cotrimoxazole is started three times weekly beginning 1 month after transplant for *Pneumocystis carinii* pneumonia prophylaxis.

Viral prophylaxis has not been well developed. In Toronto, the present schedule is directed toward herpes simplex virus and CMV. Acyclovir (800 mg orally, three times a day) and CMV-hyperimmune globulin (1 mg/kg for 8 doses) are administered prophylactically, with gancyclovir reserved for those patients who receive a CMV-positive graft. A prospective study to determine the role of CMV-hyperimmune globulin and gancyclovir in the prophylaxis schedule is presently being formulated by the Toronto Group.

The morbidity and mortality from fungal infection in lung transplant recipients are substantial. As a result, many programs routinely employ prophylactic low-dose amphotericin B. Therapeutic doses of antifungal agents are commenced immediately on discovery of fungal infection.

Aggressive use of bronchoscopy with bronchoalveolar lavage, protected brushings, and transbronchial biopsy has been employed to enable the most accurate differentiation of infection from rejection in lung transplant recipients.

In addition to receiving these procedures when clinically indicated, all patients undergo a series of scheduled postoperative surveillance procedures. Until recently, it has been difficult to determine if the incidence and severity of rejection are similar across transplantation programs because of the lack of standardized criteria. A consensus committee of pathologists has recently been convened to develop a working formulation for the standardization of nomenclature in the diagnosis of pulmonary rejection. This standardization will enable comparison of results between institutions.[28]

Patients usually remain in the intensive care unit for 24 hours after extubation, after which time they are transferred to a step-down unit.

Over the next 3 to 7 days, they are divested of their arterial line and one or more central lines. In addition, cyclosporine is switched to oral dosing, and the antilymphocyte globulin infusion is terminated. The exercise program then becomes more rigorous, and self-medication is initiated. The length of hospital stay after an uncomplicated single-lung transplant is usually 3 and a half to 5 weeks.

Once discharged from the hospital, lung transplant patients are monitored closely for the development of complications related to graft function and immunosuppressive therapy. Patients are required to live in the region for the first 3 months after transplantation. The transplant coordinator maintains close contact with all patients to insure that cyclosporine levels are adequate and that other laboratory and clinical parameters are satisfactory. Patients continue their rehabilitation program on an outpatient basis under the supervision of the physiotherapist during this 3-month interval as well. In the Toronto program, patients are readmitted to the hospital at 3, 6, 9, 12, and 18 months after transplantation, and yearly thereafter, to undergo a series of tests to assess graft function.

In Toronto, a weekly support group meets, enabling those awaiting transplantation to interact with patients already transplanted to help them better prepare for the operation. After this meeting, patients attend the transplant clinic, where those awaiting transplantation are reviewed every 3 weeks and those who have had transplantations are seen on a regularly scheduled basis.

RESULTS OF SINGLE-LUNG TRANSPLANTATION

Early postoperative morbidity is most often related to rejection and infection. Although bronchial anastomotic healing contributed to morbidity in the early experience, the new telescoping anastomotic technique appears to have eliminated this cause. Late morbidity occurs as a result of infection, chronic rejection or bronchiolitis obliterans, renal insufficiency, and lymphoproliferative disorders.

In the 1980s, uncomplicated airway healing was difficult to achieve because of, it was felt, a combination of ischemia, rejection, steroid use, inadequate preservation, and prolonged ventilation. Airway dehiscence occurred in 10 of the first 44 single-lung transplant recipients. Three of the seven patients who survived this complication developed anastomotic strictures that were successfully managed by placement of endobronchial stents for periods that ranged from 3 months to 2 years.

Patients usually suffer between one and three episodes of rejection during the first month after transplantation. Their recovery is confirmed

TABLE 6-1. Etiology of Pulmonary
Infections in Patients Who Received
Single-Lung Transplantation in Toronto,
November 1983 to March 1991

Etiology	Incidence
Bacterial	63%
Viral	25%
Fungal	10%
Pneumocystis carinii pneumonia	2%

by transbronchial biopsy about 1 week after treatment with 1 g of IV methylprednisolone daily for 3 days.

The first 44 single-lung recipients in Toronto suffered an average of 3.3 infections in the postoperative period. Bacterial pneumonia and tracheobronchitis commonly occur early (Table 6-1). Treatment is initiated with broad-spectrum antibiotics and is subsequently tailored to suit the offending organism. Cytomegalovirus pneumonitis (either primary or reactivation) is not uncommon, partly because it is not practical to insist on CMV compatibility with existing donor organ constraints. Aggressive treatment with gancyclovir is mandatory to minimize morbidity and avert mortality. The role of CMV-hyperimmune globulin has yet to be defined in the treatment of CMV infection or disease.

One of the 27 survivors of single lung transplantation in Toronto has bronchiolitis obliterans in his transplanted lung. A second patient has undergone successful retransplantation. It appears that the incidence of this complication after lung transplantation is about 10% and occurs with similar frequency as after heart–lung transplantation. While the etiology of bronchiolitis obliterans is still debated, most investigators believe that it is a manifestation of chronic rejection. Patients who suffer severe bouts of acute rejection in the early post-transplant period may be at increased risk for its development.

Lymphoproliferative disease has occurred and was fatal in one Toronto single-lung recipient. As with other solid organ transplants, a reduction in immunosuppression may effectively deal with this complication if recognized early enough.

Actuarial 1-year survival after single-lung transplantation was 51% among patients transplanted between 1983 and 1988. Patients transplanted in 1989 and 1990, however, have an actuarial 1-year survival of 68% (Fig. 6-3).

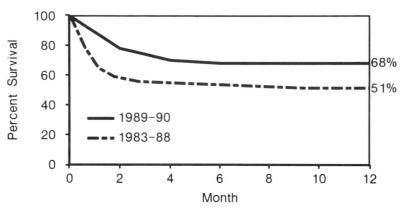

ST. LOUIS LUNG TRANSPLANT REGISTRY
SINGLE LUNG TRANSPLANTATION
1 YEAR ACTUARIAL SURVIVAL

FIGURE 6-3.   Comparison of the 1-year actuarial survival of single-lung recipients transplanted between 1983 to 1988 and 1989 to 1990. *(Courtesy of the St. Louis Lung Transplant Registry, April 1991)*

Eight early deaths occurred among the first 44 Toronto single- lung transplant recipients (Table 6-2). One death, due to air embolism, was wholly preventable, and it is felt that deaths from airway dehiscence should be eliminated with technical modifications previously discussed.

Ten late deaths occurred among the first 44 single-lung recipients. Seven deaths were secondary to infection, and one involved chronic rejection or bronchiolitis obliterans (Table 6-3). One death each occurred from renal failure and lymphoproliferative disease.

TABLE 6-2.   30-Day Mortality in Patients Who Received Single-Lung Transplantation in Toronto, November 1983 to March 1991

Cause of Death	Number of Patients
Air embolism	1
Primary graft failure	1
Airway dehiscence	3
Infection	2
Multisystem organ failure and airway dehiscence	1
Total	8 (19%)

TABLE 6-3. Late Mortality in Patients Who Received Single-Lung Transplantation in Toronto, November 1983 to March 1991

Cause of Death	Number of Patients
Infection	7
Chronic rejection or bronchiolitis obliterans	1
Renal failure	1
Lymphoproliferative disease	1
Total	10 (22.7%)
Mortality of retransplantation	50%

THE FUTURE

The recent observation that lung transplant recipients at the University of Toronto double their serum creatinine within 6 months of transplantation points to a need to alter cyclosporine administration schedules.[29] With the evidence that early steroid might not be as detrimental as once thought and the knowledge that patients who receive renal grafts do not generally receive cyclosporine for the first postoperative week, perhaps a similar modification in the cyclosporine administration schedule could be tried in lung transplant recipients.

It has been suggested that we rethink the role of cytolytic therapy (OKT3, antilymphocyte globulin) in the immunosuppression regimen based on a substantial reduction in the incidence of CMV infection and disease in patients in whom this therapy was withheld.[30]

Hypercholesterolemia related to cyclosporine administration has been relatively refractory to conventional dietary and pharmacologic therapy. The incidence of lovastatin-induced myositis is higher in immunosuppressed patients, and it is anticipated that a more acceptable lipid-lowering medication will be developed.

Heart and kidney recipients who receive no chronic steroid administration have less hypertension and a lower incidence of infection despite therapeutic levels of cyclosporine. Long-term steroid use may not be necessary and may even be harmful. Many heart–lung recipients at Papworth Hospital are not on chronic steroid therapy and have not demonstrated any ill effects from this modification in their immunosuppression. Some lung transplant surgeons feel that we are using too much immunosuppression at present. Modifications in regimens are likely to continue to occur.

Alternative forms of immunosuppression, such as FK-506, are likely to become commercially available. The risks of FK-506 in lung transplant patients have to be determined and weighed against its benefit before cyclosporine is dismissed from immunosuppression protocols. Preliminary evidence from Pittsburgh trials of FK-506 indicate that, while the risk of renal failure remains unchanged with its use, the incidence of hypertension and hypercholesterolemia might be substantially reduced with equivalent graft function and survival.[31]

While it has proved difficult to prolong the period of safe ischemia, investigation that is focusing at the molecular level promises to yield new clues into what alterations are required in present techniques of lung preservation. The use of anti-CD18 monoclonal antibody has, for example, been shown to limit ischemia–reperfusion-induced microvascular injury in a rabbit bowel model.[32]

Improvement in our ability to differentiate infection from rejection will likely develop as experience with bronchoalveolar lavage and transbronchial biopsy is gained. In addition, comparison of results between institutions will be facilitated by use of the newly developed consensus criteria for grading rejection.[28]

We are at a time of exponential growth in clinical lung transplantation and lung transplant research, and the future promises to be an exciting one.

References

1. Demikhov VP: Experimental Transplantation of Vital Organs. New York, Consultants Bureau Enterprises, 1962.
2. Metras H: Note preliminaire sur la greffe totale du puomon chez le chien. C R Acad Sci 231:1176, 1950
3. Juvenelle AA, Citret C, Wiles CE et al: Pneumonectomy with replantation of the lung in the dog for physiological study. J Thorac Surg 21:111, 1951
4. Hardy JD, Webb WR, Dalton ML et al: Lung homotransplantation in man: Report of the initial case. JAMA 186:1065, 1963
5. Wildevuur CR, Benfield JR: A review of 23 human lung transplantation by 20 surgeons. Ann Thorac Surg 9:489, 1970
6. Derom F, Barbier F, Ringoir S et al: Ten month survival after lung homotransplantation in man. J Thorac Cardiovasc Surg 61:835, 1971
7. Kaiser LR: Long-term survival statistics. Presented at the Washington University Lung Transplantation Seminar II, St. Louis, MO, October 1990
8. Novick RJ, Menkis AH, McKenzie FN et al: Prednisone is not deleterious to airway healing following lung and heart-lung transplantation (abstr). Presented at the 56th Annual Scientific Assembly ACCP, Toronto, Canada, October 1990

9. Egan TM, Kaiser LR, Cooper JD: Lung transplantation Curr Probl Surg 26:712, 1989
10. Patterson GA, Cooper JD: Status of lung transplantation. Surg Clin North Am 68:545, 1988
11. Starnes VA, Hammon JW, Lupinette FM, Olson RD, Boucek RJ Jr, Bender HW Jr: Functional and metabolic preservation of the immature myocardium with verapamil following global ischemia. Ann Thorac Surg 34:58, 1982
12. Baldwin JC, Frist WH, Starkey TD et al: Distant graft procurement for combined heart and lung transplantation using pulmonary artery flush and simple topical hypothermia for graft preservation. Ann Thorac Surg 43:670, 1987
13. Baumgartner WA, Williams GM, Fraser CD Jr et al: Cardiopulmonary bypass with profound hypothermia: An optimal method for multiorgan procurement. Transplantation 47:123, 1989
14. Novitzky D, Cooper DKC, Reichart B: Hemodynamic and metabolic responses to hormonal therapy in brain-dead potential organ donors. Transplantation 43:852, 1987
15. Hooper TL, Thomson DS, Jones MT et al: Amelioration of lung ischemic injury with prostacyclin. Transplantation 49:1031, 1990
16. Yamazaki F, Yokomise H, Keshavjee SH et al: The superiority of an extracellular fluid solution over euro-collins' solution for pulmonary preservation. Transplantation 49:690, 1990
17. Paull DE, Keagy BA, Kron EJ, Wilcox BR: Improved lung preservation using a dimethylthiourea flush. J Surg Res 46:333, 1989
18. Hachida M, Morton DL: The protection of ischemic lung with verapamil and hydralazine. J Thorac Cardiovasc Surg 95:178, 1988
19. Yokomise H, Ueno T, Yamazaki F, Keshavjee S, Slutsky A, Patterson G et al: The effect and optimal time of administration of verapamil on lung preservation. Transplantation 49:1039, 1990
20. Todd TR, Goldberg M, Koshal A et al: Separate extraction of cardiac and pulmonary grafts from a single organ donor. Ann Thorac Surg 46:356, 1988
21. DeMajo WAP: Anesthetic technique for single lung transplantation. In Cooper DKC, Novitzky D (eds): The Transplantation and Replacement of Thoracic Organs, p. 375. Boston, Kluwer Academic Publishers, 1990
22. Lima O, Cooper JD, Peters WJ et al: Effects of methylprednisolone and azathioprine on bronchial healing following lung transplantation. J Thorac Cardiovasc Surg 82:211, 1981
23. Trinkle JK, Calhoon JH, Bryan CL et al: Single lung transplantation: Alternative indications and technique (abstr). Presented at the 70th Annual Meeting of the American Association for Thoracic Surgery, Toronto, Canada, 1990
24. Pinsker RL, Koerner SK, Kamholz SL et al: Effect of donor bronchial length on healing. J Thorac Cardiovasc Surg 77:669, 1979
25. Morgan E, Lima O, Goldberg M, Ferdman A, Luk SK, Cooper JD: Successful revascularization of totally ischemic bronchial autografts with omental pedicle flaps in dogs. J Thorac Cardiovasc Surg 84:204, 1982
26. Veith FJ, Richards K: Improved technique for canine lung transplantation. Ann Surg 171:553, 1970

27. Waters P, Ross D, Trento A et al: Experience with OKT3 in heart–lung transplantation (abstr). Presented at the 56th Annual Scientific Assembly ACCP, Toronto, Canada, October 1990
28. Berry GJ, Brunt EM, Chamberlain D et al: A working formulation for the standardization of nomenclature in the diagnosis of heart and lung rejection: lung rejection study group. J Heart Transplant 9:593, 1990
29. Zaltzman JS, Pei Y, Maurer J et al: Cyclosporine A (CyA) nephrotoxicity in lung transplant recipients (abstr). Presented at the University of Toronto Day in Transplantation, 1990
30. Trinkle JK, Calhoon JH, Nichols L et al: Single lung transplantation: Factors in postoperative infections (abstr). Presented at the 57th Annual Assembly AATS, Washington, DC, 1990
31. Starzl TE, Abu-Elmagd K, Tzakis A, Fung JJ, Porter KA, Todo S: Selected topics on FK-506 with specific reference to rescue of extrahepatic whole organ grafts, transplantation of forbidden organs, side effects, mechanisms and practical pharmacology. Transplant Proc 23:914, 1991
32. Hernandez LA, Grisham MB, Twohig B, Arfors KE, Harlan JN, Granger DN: Role of neutrophils in ischemia–reperfusion-induced microvascular injury. Am J Physiol 253:H699, 1987

Simon Gelman
Yoo Goo Kang
James D. Pearson

7 Anesthetic Considerations in Liver Transplantation

A valuable alternative to patients with irreversible end-stage liver disease whose life expectancy would otherwise be short is liver transplantation. A large number of patients have undergone liver transplantation and now enjoy normal productive lives; some patients have even had successful pregnancies. Improvements in outcome and decreases in morbidity have been achieved through improved surgical techniques and donor-organ preservation and through availability of less toxic and more effective immunosuppressive drugs.

The broad indications for hepatic transplantation in adults include end-stage cirrhosis (e.g., primary biliary cirrhosis, chronic active hepatitis, cryptogenic cirrhosis, secondary biliary cirrhosis, autoimmune cirrhosis, primary sclerosing cholangitis), fulminant hepatic failure, and metabolic disorders such as Wilson's disease, protoporphyria, hemochromatosis, type IV hyperlipidemia, Budd-Chiari syndrome, primary hepatocellular carcinoma, and others. Liver transplantation in children is performed for end-stage cirrhosis (e.g., biliary atresia , extrahepatic as well as intrahepatic, congenital biliary cirrhosis, congenital hepatic fibrosis, chronic active hepatitis), metabolic disorders (e.g., alpha$_1$-antitrypsin deficiency, tyrosinemia, galactosemia, glycogen storage disease, types I and IV), familial cholestasis, sea-blue histiocyte syndrome, and others. It has been shown that children usually do better than adults, and patients with cholestatic disease do better than those with parenchymal hepatic disease.[1]

Knowledge of the pathophysiology of the underlying disease is extremely important for planning and providing adequate and justified anesthesia and intensive care for any patient, particularly those with complicated hemodynamic, pulmonary, and metabolic disorders, such as patients with end-stage hepatic disease. Therefore, the following section highlights the most important characteristics of patients with end-stage hepatic disease who might undergo hepatic transplantation.

ANATOMY AND PHYSIOLOGY OF THE LIVER

The liver was defined as an acinus by Rappaport and associates more than 20 years ago.[2] According to their idea, hepatocytes are grouped into three zones that surround the terminal afferent vessels (Fig. 7-1). Zone 1 cells are in close proximity to the terminal vessels and receive blood first. They are also the first to regenerate and the last to develop necrosis. Zones 2 and 3 receive blood that contains smaller amounts of oxygen and nutritives and consequently do not withstand hepatotoxins, oxygen deprivation, and other damaging factors.

The blood supply of the liver is twofold (Fig. 7–2). Hepatic blood flow is about 100 mL/min/100 g, which represents about 25% of cardiac output; 65% to 80% of total hepatic blood flow is supplied by the portal veins, and the remaining 20% to 35% is supplied by the hepatic artery. More oxygen is found in hepatic arterial blood than in portal blood, and, therefore, the hepatic arterial blood provides nearly 50% of the total oxygen delivered and consumed. The liver contains about 20 to 30 mL of blood per 100 g of liver tissue, representing about 15% of total blood volume. In conditions of increased sympathetic tone, half of this volume can be mobilized, thereby demonstrating that the liver is a major blood reservoir.

The arterioles in the preportal splanchnic organs mainly control portal venous blood flow. This flow, together with the resistance to flow in the preportal vasculature and, to an extent, within the liver, establishes portal pressure (7–10 mm Hg). The relatively unchanging distribution of flow through the liver is determined by the presinusoidal (precapillary) sphincters, which also function (to a limited extent) in the regulation of portal blood flow; however, it appears that postsinusoidal resistance is an important site of venous resistance within the liver. The tone of presinusoidal and postsinusoidal sphincters and blood flow determines sinusoidal pressure. Smooth muscle in the wall of the venules regulates

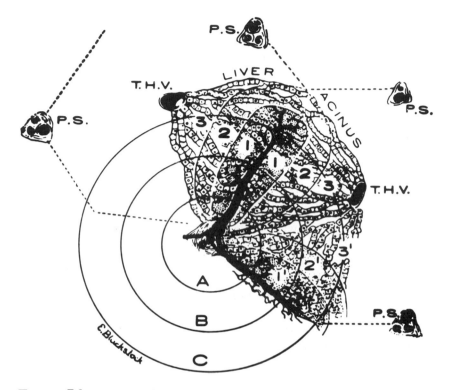

FIGURE 7-1. The blood supply of the hepatic structural unit: the structural unit occupies adjacent sectors of neighboring hexagonal fields. Zones 1, 2, and 3 represent areas supplied with blood of first, second, and third quality, respectively, with regard to oxygen and nutrients. These zones cluster about the terminal afferent vascular twigs and extend into the periportal field from which these twigs originate. Zones 1', 2', and 3' designate corresponding areas in a portion of an adjacent structural unit. In zones 1 and 1', the afferent vascular twigs empty into the sinusoids. The circles *A, B,* and *C* delimit concentric bands of the hepatic parenchyma arranged around a small portal field. *PS,* portal space; *THV,* terminal hepatic venules. *(Rappaport AM, Borowy ZJ, Lougheed WM, Lotto WN: Subdivision of hexagonal liver lobules into a structural and functional unit. Anat Rec 119:16, 1954)*

venous compliance and blood volume. Both resistance and compliance in the portal venous vasculature are primarily controlled by sympathetic innervation mediated through α-adrenergic receptors. Cardiac output is largely controlled by changes in hepatic venous compliance. Hepatic venous resistance is an important mechanism that regulates both portal pressure and trans-sinusoidal fluid movements. Myogenic and metabolic intrinsic regulation play a little role, if any, in controlling hepatic venous

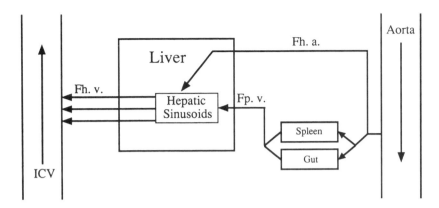

FIGURE 7-2.   Schematic representation of liver blood supply. ICV equals inferior caval vein; Fh.v., hepatic venous flow; Fh.a., hepatic arterial flow; Fp.v., portal venous flow.

resistance. Sympathetic innervation mediated via α-adrenergic receptors appears to be the main mechanism responsible for the regulation of hepatic venous capacitance. The sinusoids are relatively permeable to protein. As sinusoidal pressure increases, filtration of fluid increases, and protein passes more readily into the lymph vessels.

PATHOPHYSIOLOGY OF LIVER DISEASE

End-stage hepatic disease is often associated with an increase in portal venous pressure, a reduction in portal venous blood flow, an increase in portal-systemic shunting, and a decrease in peripheral vascular resistance and arterial pressure with a subsequent increase in cardiac output.

The pathogenesis of portal hypertension is rather complex. The classic "backward theory" regards portal hypertension to be a result of liver cirrhosis (fibrosis) with a subsequent increase in resistance to portal flow. However, experimentally induced restriction to portal flow is not usually accompanied by an increase in portal pressure and is rarely associated with bleeding from esophageal varices. More importantly, experimentally induced restriction to portal flow is often concomitant with a decrease in mesenteric flow, an increase in mesenteric vascular resistance, an immediate decrease in oxygen content in portal blood, and an increase in arteriovenous oxygen content difference, contrary to the pattern found in cirrhotic patients. The so-called "forward theory" of portal hypertension suggests that some factors lead to vasodilation and the formation of arteriovenous fistulas in the gut and spleen with an increased splanchnic flow and the development of a hyperdynamic state.[3,4] As an interesting point, the first study that suggested the "forward theory" was published at the beginning of this century. In 1904, Kretz demonstrated arteriovenous communications with "arterial mixture in the portal vein" in portal hypertension.[5] An increase in splanchnic flow and an increase in resistance to portal flow are apparently responsible for the well-known clinical picture of portal hypertension.[6]

Multiple factors lead to splanchnic vasodilation. In patients with liver cirrhosis, glucagon concentrations are increased. Moreover, the increase in glucagon concentrations parallels the increase in blood ammonia concentrations.[7] In rats in which portal hypertension was experimentally induced, the increased glucagon concentration was responsible for 40% of the mesenteric vascular resistance decrease and mesenteric flow increase.[8] The remaining 60% of the observed decrease in mesenteric vascular resistance may be attributed to other vasodilating substances, such as vasoactive intestinal polypeptide or ferritin.[9,10]

In patients with liver cirrhosis and portal hypertension, the concentrations of many vasoconstricting substances are increased. Norepinephrine and epinephrine concentrations were found to be 314% and 280% of controls, respectively.[11] Increased norepinephrine concentrations correlated positively with the occluded hepatic venous pressure (which reflects portal venous pressure) and inversely correlated with plasma volume. It is interesting that sensitivity to norepinephrine is substantially diminished in portal hypertension.[12] Since glucagon serves as an antagonist to the vasoconstricting effects of hepatic nerve stimulation and norepinephrine infusion, increased glucagon concentrations can be responsible for this decrease in sensitivity to norepinephrine.[13] In patients with liver cirrhosis and portal hypertension, a definite correlation has also been found between the occluded hepatic vein pressure and plasma renin activity.[14]

CARDIOPULMONARY SEQUELAE OF LIVER DISEASE

Patients with liver cirrhosis and portal hypertension are usually in a hyperdynamic state with decreased vascular resistance and arterial blood pressure and increased cardiac output. If arterial hypotension results from hypovolemia because of hemorrhage or increased capillary permeability, calculated peripheral vascular resistance would increase. Increased concentrations of circulating vasoactive substances such as glucagon, vasoactive intestinal polypeptide, ferritin, and others are largely responsible for the reduced peripheral vascular resistance in liver disease, especially if they are associated with liver cirrhosis and portal hypertension. Several important determinants in the pathogenesis of the reduced vascular resistance are seen: an increase in arteriovenous shunting, a decrease in sensitivity to catecholamines, and abnormal plasma concentrations of prostaglandins. These patients have an increased venous oxygen saturation and a decreased arteriovenous oxygen content difference. Despite the increased cardiac output, hepatic blood flow is reduced in liver cirrhosis as a result of a drastic reduction in portal blood flow. Hepatic arterial blood flow is maintained or even increased. A high cardiac output is possible because of the low peripheral vascular resistance with subsequent increases in stroke volume, despite the cardiomyopathy with impaired myocardial contractility that is often seen in patients with cirrhosis. An early predictor of cardiac decompensation in cirrhotic patients is an increased heart rate without other associated medical problems, such as bleeding or pulmonary dysfunction. Ascites per se can jeopardize the cardiovascular system by increasing intra-abdominal and intrathoracic pressures with an associated decrease in venous return.

The majority of patients with liver cirrhosis and portal hypertension are hypoxemic. A reduction in arterial oxygen content may result from the following: intrapulmonary shunt, ventilation–perfusion abnormalities, alveolar hypoventilation (which results from ascites), decreased pulmonary diffusing capacity, and a shift in the oxygen-hemoglobin dissociation curve to the right (decreased affinity of oxygen for hemoglobin).

Intrapulmonary shunt (venous admixture) in patients with portal hypertension is due to shunting of venous blood through arteriovenous fistulas similar to spider angiomas seen on the skin. Also, certain vascular communications occur between the portal veins and pulmonary veins through azygos, mediastinal, and periesophageal veins. Patients with cirrhosis do not increase their pulmonary vascular resistance while breathing a low oxygen mixture. Therefore, it is suggested by these and other data that hypoxic pulmonary vasoconstriction is impaired in these patients, resulting in a ventilation–perfusion mismatch with a subsequent decrease in arterial oxygen content. Intrapulmonary vasodilation is also related to increased glucagon and vasoactive intestinal polypeptide concentrations in patients with liver disease.

Another cause of hypoxemia is alveolar hypoventilation, which can be attributed to ascites and to an increased intra-abdominal pressure with a decrease in pulmonary functional residual capacity. Pulmonary diffusing capacity can also be impaired secondary to an increase in extracellular fluid. The reduction in the affinity of hemoglobin for oxygen leads to different degrees of arterial oxygen desaturation. This reduced

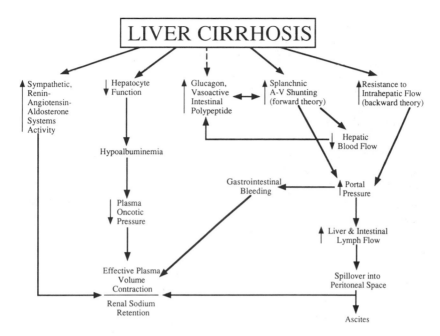

FIGURE 7-3.   Schematic representation of pathogenesis of liver cirrhosis.

affinity is caused by metabolic acidosis, which sometimes develops in patients with liver disease. The pathogenesis of hypoxemia in patients with liver cirrhosis is schematically represented in Figure 7-3.

Cardiopulmonary dysfunction in patients with liver disease often does not require special vigorous measures. Pharmacologic and ventilatory support is sometimes required in the terminal stages of liver disease.

RENAL DYSFUNCTION AND HEPATORENAL SYNDROME

The development of renal dysfunction in patients with liver failure is not completely understood. One of the most important features of renal dysfunction in patients with advanced liver disease is the primary (partially due to increased levels of aldosterone) or secondary (due to reduced "effective" plasma volume) renal tubular retention and reabsorption of sodium. The decrease in effective plasma volume (due mainly to the redistribution of fluid from the intravascular to interstitial space and ascites) is unavoidably accompanied by the activation of volume receptors with subsequent increases in sympathetic nervous activity and angiotensin concentrations, renin release, aldosterone secretion, and intrarenal blood flow redistribution. Increased adrenal secretion, as well as decreased metabolic degradation of the hormone, is responsible for the elevated plasma concentration of aldosterone. The rate of hepatic deterioration of aldosterone is primarily related to hepatic blood flow. This flow is significantly reduced in the majority of patients with severe liver disease, particularly cirrhosis.

Water diuresis is also impaired in patients with liver disease. Enhanced antidiuretic hormone (ADH) activity is largely accountable for water retention as well as the decreased delivery to filtrate the diluting segments of the nephron. Increased ADH concentration results in augmented back-diffusion of free water in the collecting tubules. Most likely, increased ADH concentration in patients with liver disease is mediated through nonosmotic stimuli, including a decrease in peripheral vascular resistance and arterial pressure. Impaired metabolic clearance of ADH-vasopressin also contributes to increased ADH activity. After gastrointestinal bleeding and hypotension, dehydration and absorption of large amounts of nitrogenous substances from the gut can also contribute to renal dysfunction. Even severe renal dysfunction is often reversible, but sometimes renal lesions can be serious, including acute tubular necrosis. Characteristics of reversible renal dysfunction in patients with hepatic disease include normal urinary sediment and urinary sodium concentrations of less than 20 mM^{-1}. Serum creatinine concentrations are a much better index for determining the extent of renal impairment than blood urea concentrations, since hepatic failure is sometimes associated with a decrease in the rate of urea synthesis in the liver.

It appears that renal failure in the hepatorenal syndrome is functional in nature. Pathologic abnormalities are minimal and inconsistent despite severe renal dysfunction. Tubular functional integrity is manifested by relatively unimpaired concentrating ability. Normal renal function resumes in recipients of kidney transplants harvested from patients with hepatorenal syndrome. However, the pathogenesis of the hepatorenal syndrome still remains unknown. During the development of the hepatorenal syndrome, renal hemodynamic disorders, along with a particular reduction in cortical perfusion and the evolvement of intrarenal shunts,[15] play an important, if not crucial, role. Other factors involved in this pathogenesis are activation of the renin-angiotensin system, an increase in sympathetic nervous activity, alterations in the endogenous release of renal prostaglandins, changes in the kallikrein-kinin system, increased levels of vasoactive intestinal polypeptide, and other vasoactive compounds.

The renin activity, aldosterone, and norepinephrine concentrations have been substantially increased—twofold to fivefold—in patients with liver cirrhosis without renal failure when compared to healthy controls. When renal failure developed, these concentrations doubled or even tripled. The concentrations of some prostaglandins (PGE_2) and kallikreins in urine were two times higher in patients with liver cirrhosis without renal failure than in healthy controls. However, these values decreased from 50% to 25% of controls when renal failure developed.[16] Renal plasma flow and glomerular filtration rate were obviously much lower in cirrhotic patients with renal failure than in patients without renal failure. Prostaglandins (PGE_2) and kallikreins play a compensatory protective role during the decline of renal function, which is directly related to an increase in renin activity, aldosterone, and norepinephrine concentrations. Renal decompensation develops when these protective mechanisms are depleted.

Patients who present clinically with hepatorenal syndrome usually have ascites, indications of increased sodium or water retention (hypernatremia or hyponatremia), and increased renin and aldosterone activity without any indications of kidney damage (no salt waste, no hyposthenuria). Treatment of hepatorenal syndrome should include proper fluid load (preferably monitored by measurements of filling pressures), which consists of albumin, fresh frozen plasma (in patients with documented coagulopathy and bleeding), and crystalloids with an appropriate concentration of sodium (often hyponatremic or sodium-free solutions). Diuretic therapy is also important and includes furosemide, mannitol, and spironolactone. Dopamine in small doses (0.5–3 $\mu g/kg/min$) appears to be helpful. The beneficial effect of dopamine might be due to its antialdosterone effect,[17] as well as to its effect on the renal circulation. The antialdosterone effect results in improved tubular solute transport (sodium and water excretion), while hemodynamic effects are presented by vasodilation within the kidneys and, to a certain extent, an increase in cardiac output. The hepatorenal syndrome is treated most effectively by the surgical formation of a peritoneojugular shunt. The pathogenesis and treatment of renal dysfunction in patients with liver disease have been reviewed recently.[15]

Other metabolic disorders include electrolyte and acid–base imbalance, hypoglycemia, hepatic encephalopathy, and coagulopathy. The latter predisposes to hemorrhage. Coagulopathy results from thrombocytopenia and reduced plasma concentrations of liver-produced clotting factors. Thrombocytopenia is due to bone marrow depression, hypersplenism (especially in viral hepatitis), and disseminated intravascular coagulation.[18]

The liver synthesizes the following clotting factors: I (fibrinogen), II (prothrombin), V, VII, IX, and X. Hepatic failure is associated with a decrease in the synthesis of these factors, resulting in a prolonged pro-

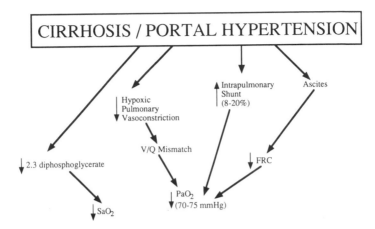

FIGURE 7-4. Schematic representation of hypoxemia in liver cirrhosis and portal hypertension. SaO_2 = arterial oxygen saturation, V/Q = ventilation/perfusion, FRC = functional residual capacity.

thrombin time (PT) and partial thromboplastin time (PTT). The extent of liver dysfunction can usually be determined by changes in PT. Factors II, VII, IX, and X are vitamin-K dependent, while factors I and V are not. Factor VIII, which is not synthesized in the liver, can be increased during liver failure. Factor VII has a relatively short half-life; therefore, it decreases sooner, probably to a greater extent than any other liver-produced clotting factor.[19] Fibrinogen (factor I) synthesis deteriorates the least. Some data indicate that the rate of fibrinogen degradation and consumption may be enhanced in hepatic failure. Heparin administration can partially help correct the abnormal metabolism of fibrinogen.[20] These data suggest the possible development of disseminated intravascular coagulation with secondary fibrinolysis in hepatic failure. Coagulopathy in hepatic failure has been recently reviewed.[21,22]

Certain dysfunctions of almost all organs and systems are a result of the complexity in the development of portal hypertension (Fig. 7-4).

PHARMACOKINETIC IMPLICATIONS OF LIVER DISEASE

Polar groups to hydrophobic molecules are added by a mixed function oxidase system (phase I). Then, by conjugating a more hydrophilic molecule to the polar group (phase II), they make these xenobiotics more water soluble and more easily excreted. In general, phase I reactions are inhibited by liver disease, while phase II reactions are reasonably well preserved.[23] The phase II or conjugating reactions are unique in that they terminate biologic activity, enhance water solubility, and aid in excretion, especially via the biliary system.

Liver dysfunction also affects drug metabolism. Higher serum concentrations of the unbound, active drugs are a result of an increased volume of distribution that is modified by fewer protein-binding sites. Decreased hepatic metabolism also plays a role, especially with drugs that undergo extensive hepatic metabolism before excretion. This process results in increased initial dose requirements as well as in prolonged elimination of many drugs.

Unfortunately, studies related to the pharmacologic effect of drugs (pharmacodynamics) in patients with hepatic disease have attracted little attention. Pharmacokinetic data would also have to be included in these studies to determine whether or not an observed effect is the result of an adjustment in the pharmacodynamics or pharmacokinetics of the drug. Altered interaction between drug and receptor (pharmacodynamics) must be differentiated from a change in the concentration of the drug available to the receptor (pharmacokinetics).

In spite of these problems, certain drugs have been studied carefully in patients with end-stage liver disease. Plasma morphine sulfate concentrations show a double-peak pattern, with the second peak occurring 4 to 5 hours after administration, that is not accounted for by intrahepatic bile circulation because the bile of these patients was drained via a T-tube.[24] Patients with severe hepatic disease and hepatic coma are much more sensitive to morphine and diazepam, possibly secondary to an alteration in the blood–brain barrier.[25,26] A significant delay in eliminating midazolam is seen in patients with severe hepatic cirrhosis.[27] Elimination half-life is not prolonged for thiopental sodium because the total plasma clearance and total apparent volume of distribution at the steady state remain virtually unchanged for thiopental sodium in patients with hepatic cirrhosis.[28] However, an increase in the unbound fraction of thiopental sodium may enhance the activity of a single dose of the drug and therefore may increase the incidence of hypotension during anesthesia induction.

Plasma clearance of fentanyl citrate is significantly decreased in patients with hepatic cirrhosis. Higher bilirubin concentrations are associated with prolonged elimination of fentanyl citrate.[29] Alfentanil also exerts a prolonged and pronounced effect in patients with advanced liver disease.[30]

Twenty years ago, it was demonstrated that higher doses of d-tubocurarine were needed to achieve a similar degree of muscle relaxation in patients with hepatic cirrhosis compared to patients with normal liver function.[31] The effect has been attributed to an increase in volume of distribution secondary to an increase in the gamma-globulin fraction of serum protein with a subsequent increase in binding of d-tubocurarine to gamma globulin and a decrease in free fraction of the drug. Pancuronium bromide elimination is also prolonged. The time to peak effect of vecuronium is significantly prolonged; however, no change in the duration of action occurs.[32] The pharmacokinetics of vecuronium are not significantly altered, and the authors have been unable to explain this effect. Atracurium in patients with acute hepatic failure has clearance and elimination half-lives similar to those observed in healthy patients, but distribution half-lives and distribution volumes are smaller in healthy patients.[33]

The lesson is clear: because of pharmacodynamic and pharmacokinetic alterations, the response of each patient to a particular drug is virtually unpredictable. Therefore, each drug must be carefully selected and, more important, must be carefully titrated to desired effect.

ANESTHETIC MANAGEMENT

Preoperative Assessment

Patients for liver transplantation present a broad range of pathophysiologic changes. The patient with postnecrotic cirrhosis may have several organ diseases and poor hepatic function, while the patient with primary hepatoma may be relatively healthy with well-preserved hepatic function. Thorough preoperative assessment of the transplant recipient is mandatory because of multiple organ involvement in end-stage liver disease. On admission for the initial screening, a complete examination of all organ systems of the transplant candidate is routinely performed. The urgency of surgery may preclude a lengthy assessment immediately before surgery. If the patient has correctable disease, attempts should be made to optimize his or her condition. Patients with severely abnormal cardiopulmonary function should be discouraged from undergoing surgery because this condition greatly increases surgical morbidity and mortality. Nevertheless, liver transplantation may be the only chance for survival.

After all of the physicians involved in the patient's care, including the anesthesiologists, have weighed the benefits and risks of surgery, the decision for transplantation is made. The patient and family should be informed of anesthetic care, postoperative care, and the risk of anesthesia and surgery at this time. When a donor organ has been located for the patient, a second visit is made to reassess the patient's current physical status. Information obtained from the previous visit is compared with current information. All consent forms should be reviewed. Frequently, the consent of both the recipient and the family is required because of the questionable mental status of the recipient.

Because of poor physical status and encephalopathy in these patients, light premedication is usually recommended. An antacid may be included in the premedication, especially when the recipient has had recent oral intake, since gastric emptying time is frequently prolonged.

It is imperative to evaluate the degree of cardiopulmonary, hepatic, renal, and other dysfunctions. Disturbances in electrolyte balance as well as the function of the coagulation system should be determined and corrected to the greatest possible extent. It is not surprising that PT and activated PTT are prolonged, and concentrations of all coagulation factors except fibrinogen and factor VIII are decreased preoperatively in patients who receive liver transplants. Although fibrinogen concentration is generally normal or even high, dysfibrinogenemia has been known to occur in patients with liver disease. This condition is indicated by a moderately prolonged thrombin time and reptilase time. The clinical significance of the acquired dysfibrinogenemia in patients who are receiving liver transplants is not known. Factor VIII concentration increases because of increased production related to stress response, release from damaged cells, or impaired biotransformation of factor VIII.[34] Platelet count is generally low, resulting from sequestration secondary to hypersplenism. In addition, abnormal platelet function may be related to a preponderance of small, hypofunctional platelets.[35] Fibrinolytic activity is increased, presumably because of defective synthesis of fibrinolytic inhibitors or delayed removal of plasminogen activators. Fibrin degradation products are positive in one third of recipients, and euglobulin lysis time is frequently less than 1 hour. Disseminated intravascular coagulation plays a controversial role. A patient with chronic liver disease may have a defective vascular phase of hemostasis, although this process is not well understood. In addition, frequent upper gastrointestinal tract bleeding from esophageal varices requires multiple preoperative transfusions, and dilutional coagulopathy may occur. The preoperative coagulation profile is scored by disease group, and the score is compared with the blood products used during liver transplantation.[36] More blood products were transfused in patients with postnecrotic cirrhosis, sclerosing cholangitis, and acute fulminant hepatitis, and the degree of hepatocellular damage appeared to be positively associated with blood transfusion volume.

In assessing the coagulation system and for anticipating the magnitude of intraoperative blood transfusion, a complete preoperative coagulation profile is useful. It might not be practical to correct the coagulation system preoperatively. Vitamin K, which is given to candidates for transplantation, does not always improve coagulation. Although blood products may be given preoperatively, the transfused blood products may be destroyed or may not function in the presence of the diseased liver. Preparation time may not be allowed because of the urgency of surgery, and exchange transfusion in the absence of hemodynamic monitoring may interfere with cardiopulmonary performance. Therefore, correction of the coagulation system is often most effective when accomplished intraoperatively.

Anemia (hematocrit less than 30%) is often seen. It may be microcytic hypochromic anemia due to gastrointestinal bleeding or macrocytic anemia from folic acid deficiency.

Blood glucose concentration should be determined preoperatively and hypoglycemia or hyperglycemia appropriately corrected.

The preoperative evaluation should include the possibility of transmission of hepatitis. Hepatitis screening should be performed to protect other surgical patients and health care personnel. Personnel should take precautions to not be contaminated by hepatitis, and all patients with a history of hepatitis are regarded as infective unless the absence of antigenemia is proven.

Monitoring and Preparation

A summary of the anesthetic management for liver transplantation appears in Appendix 7.1. The successful conclusion of surgery and uneventful recovery dependent on aggressive monitoring and proper interpretation of the monitored variables. The cardiovascular system is usually monitored by electrocardiography, radial arterial pressure, central venous pressure, pulmonary arterial pressure, and cardiac output, determined by thermodilution technique. Serial measurements of arterial blood gas tensions and end-tidal CO_2 tension are also included. Hourly urine output and urine specific gravity measurements are beneficial in assessing renal function. Body temperature is monitored by measuring rectal, esophageal, and blood temperatures. The laboratory determinations needed during surgery are arterial blood gas tensions and acid–base state, hemoglobin concentration, hematocrit level, and serum concentrations of sodium, potassium, ionized calcium, and glucose. These are measured hourly or more frequently, when needed. Finally, the blood coagulation system is evaluated by means of the PT, activated

PTT, and platelet count; determination of thrombin time, reptilase time, plasma clot lysis time, levels of factors I, II, and VIII, fibrin split products, results of the ethanol gel test, and euglobulin lysis time are also helpful. Thromboelastography has been helpful in assessing function of the blood coagulation system at the bedside.[37,38]

Particular attention should be paid to establishing adequate intravenous (IV) access to use one of the rapid infusion systems. The patient should be positioned during preparation for surgery by using foam padding to protect the sacrum and heels, and minimize brachial plexus tension.

Intraoperative Anesthetic Management

Anesthesia induction is well tolerated in most patients without serious cardiac disease. All patients should be considered to have a full stomach because gastric emptying time can be prolonged and urgency of surgery might not allow enough time for gastric emptying. Preoxygenation followed by rapid induction with cricoid pressure is usually used. Anesthesia induction is achieved with sodium pentothal or, in some cases, ketamine. Controlled normoventilation is provided, and positive end-expiratory pressure (5 cm H_2O) is added to the ventilatory circuit. FIO_2 is maintained between 0.5 and 0.7. Prolonged exposure to nitrous oxide might distend the bowels, thereby making the surgical closure of the abdomen difficult and possibly increasing the size of air emboli.[39] Therefore, nitrous oxide is usually not administered. The combination of isoflurane and fentanyl citrate is probably advantageous, since experimental evidence strongly suggests that these two anesthetics provide the optimal hepatic oxygen supply–demand relationship and protection from ischemic insult.[40,41] A long-acting nondepolarizing muscle relaxant is usually used during the liver transplantation.

Hepatic transplantation can be divided into four stages: hepatectomy, anhepatic stage, reperfusion, and neohepatic or biliary reconstruction. The first stage, hepatectomy, lasts from the beginning of the surgery until all vessels (hepatic artery, portal vein, and inferior caval vein below and above the liver) are clamped and the liver is removed. The main problems observed during this stage include bleeding, which is sometimes quite severe because of increased splanchnic flow, arteriovenous shunts, and adhesions. Cardiovascular changes may result not only from bleeding but also from the compression of the inferior vena cava and pericardium with a subsequent decrease in venous return. Renal function should be carefully monitored, and proper volume and diuretics should be administered, if needed, in this and subsequent stages of liver transplantation. Function of the coagulation system should also be monitored by relatively frequent thromboelastograms, as well as determination of PT, PTT, fibrinogen, platelets, and other components of the coagulation system. Treatment should be provided according to the results and should usually include infusion of fresh frozen plasma, platelets, and cryoprecipitate. A detailed description of the management of the coagulopathy during hepatic transplantation can be found elsewhere.[42]

Decreases in body temperature often occur during this and subsequent stages of hepatectomy. Use of a humidifier with warm gases, blankets, nasogastric lavage with warm saline, and even intra-abdominal administration of warm saline may be needed. When hyperkalemia occurs, diuresis (dopamine 2–3 μg/kg/min, furosemide, mannitol) and proper fluid replacement with solutions that do not contain potassium (D_5W in case of hypernatremia or saline otherwise), as well as the use of calcium, glucose and insulin, and sodium bicarbonate, may be needed. At the end of this stage, porto-femoral-axillary bypass begins. This procedure is associated with an increase in flow through the superior vena caval system and often results in increases in the central venous and pulmonary arterial pressures. Air embolism may occur during this time. Low flow through the bypass apparatus suggests kinked tubing, thrombosis, or hypovolemia. In normal adults, flow is usually 1 to 4 L/min.

The second or anhepatic stage of liver transplantation begins with removal of the liver and includes inferior vena caval (both above and below the liver) and portal venous vascular anastomoses. Some surgeons include hepatic arterial anastomosis in this stage, while others prefer to construct the hepatic arterial anastomosis after reperfusion (the next stage). Thus, the stage lasts until these three or four anastomoses are completed. The anhepatic stage is often associated with metabolic acidosis (treated with sodium bicarbonate), citrate intoxication (which can be suggested by hemodynamic changes), and changes in QT intervals on the electrocardiogram (usually treated with IV administration of calcium). Coagulopathy, hypothermia, and hyperpotassemia are treated as in the previous stage. At the very end of the anhepatic stage, calcium chloride (1–2 g) and sodium bicarbonate (50 mEq) are usually administered.

The reperfusion stage (third stage) begins with the unclamping of the vessels and lasts until biliary construction starts. This stage of hepatic transplantation can be associated with the most dramatic metabolic and hemodynamic disturbances. In 30% of patients, so-called "postreperfusion syndrome" develops during this stage. The syndrome consists of hypotension, bradycardia, decreased cardiac output and systemic vascular resistance, and increased filling pressures. The pathophysiology of reperfusion syndrome is complex, not well understood, and more than likely includes hyperpotassemia, metabolic acidosis, sudden decreases in body temperature by 0.5 to 1.5°C, air embolism, right ventricular overload, and influence of cardiodepressant and vasoactive substances washed out from the new liver (e.g., prostaglandins, kallikreins, platelet activation factors, leukotrienes). Treatment of this stage usually includes administration of calcium, sodium bicarbonate, glucose and insulin, and atropine (in case of severe bradycardia). Preload should be optimized, usually by fluid restriction at this time if severe bleeding does not occur. Occasionally, injection of epinephrine (10 μg boluses or an infusion) may be required. Hyperglycemia can develop late in this period and particularly during the following stage (biliary construction). The pathogenesis of hyperglycemia is not clear but may result, at least partially, from impaired glucose use in the tissues.

The fourth and last stage of liver transplantation (neohepatic or biliary reconstruction) begins with biliary reconstruction and lasts until the end of the surgical procedure. Usually the anesthesiologist does not encounter many problems during this stage. However, coagulopathy and bleeding (due to coagulopathy or insufficient surgical hemostasis) can occur. Abdominal closure may present problems secondary to bowel distention, which is due to circulatory disturbances and edema in the splanchnic organs and tissues. Since veno-venous bypass has been introduced, such difficulties are minimized; they can be quite dramatic, however, if surgery is prolonged and bypass is not used.

Successful completion of this stage allows entrance into the challenging arena of the postoperative period, which encompasses all of the features of the healing process in critically ill patients and is complicated by the ever-present risk of organ rejection and infection.

APPENDIX: LIVER TRANSPLANT PROTOCOL

Anesthetic Preparation

I. Machine
   A. Usual set-up and position
   B. Add Pall filters to both inspiratory and expiratory limbs of circuit
   C. Add 5-cm PEEP valve to expiratory limb
   D. Add Fisher/Paykel circuit humidifier with special hoses; fill with 250 mL sterile water

II. Monitors
   A. Electrocardiography: all leads on back; cover each with bio-occlusive dressing
   B. Noninvasive blood pressure: to right arm
   C. Temperature: monitored by automatic Foley catheter and by blood temperature with pulmonary artery catheter
   D. Gas monitor: Datex 254
   E. Urine output: automatic Foley catheter
   F. Arterial line: right radial artery, 18-g catheter preferred
   G. Pulmonary artery catheter: oximetric, regular
   H. Pulse oximeter: right hand
III. Intravenous Access/Fluids
   A. Lines
      1. 16-g or 14-g peripheral IV right arm, connected to fluid warmer (optional)
      2. Two 8.5 F introducers in right internal jugular; insert two guide wires then place introducers
         a. Attach one of the introducers to rapid infuser; remove valve-sideport attachment and connect directly to introducer to decrease resistance
         b. Introduce pulmonary artery catheter via second introducer
         c. Sideport is used for drug administration (e.g., dopamine); may use D_5W with microdrip as carrier solution, run through multiple stopcock manifold
      3. 9F introducer in left upper arm, basilic vein, sutured in; may use for fluids; will be used with special connector for veno-venous bypass
IV. Additional Equipment
   Sterile gloves, PEEP valves 5, 7.5, 10, 12.5 cm H_2O, automatic Foley catheter, nasogastric tube (careful insertion to prevent bleeding) foam headrest, foam padding for arms and to place under sacrum and heels, egg crate mattress, warming blanket (38°C), fluid bag (500–1,000 mL) to place between arm and steel frame for padding to prevent nerve injury, autotransfuser (BRAT) may be needed
V. Available Drugs
   A. For anesthesia
      1. Thiopental sodium, ketamine, midazolam
      2. Succinylcholine, vecuronium, or pancuronium bromide
      3. O_2, air, isoflurane
      4. Fentanyl citrate (may need up to 50 µg/kg) 20-mL vials

B. Infusions
   1. Dopamine, 400 mg/250 mL D_5W, begin at 2.5 $\mu g/kg/min$
   2. Phenylephrine, 10 mg/250 mL
   3. Nitroglycerin, 50 mg/250 mL
   4. Be prepared to mix epinephrine 1 mg/250 mL
C. Syringes for boluses
   1. Ephedrine, 5 mg/mL
   2. Atropine, 0.8 mg/mL
   3. Lidocaine, 100 mg/mL
   4. Epinephrine, 10 $\mu g/mL$ (1 ampule diluted to 10 mL)
   5. $NaHCO_3$
   6. $CaCl_2$
D. Miscellaneous
   1. Mannitol
   2. Furosemide
   3. Imipenem-cilastatin sodium, 500 mg/250 mL IV every 6 hours
   4. Epsilon Aminocaproic acid (EACA), 1 g IV if needed for fibrinolysis during neohepatic phase
   5. Hydrocortisone 1 g
   6. Lactated Ringer's solution 1000 mL refrigerated, to flush donor liver before reperfusion
   7. Insulin
   8. $D_{50}W$

Stages of Anesthesia and Operation

I. Anesthetic Induction
   A. Position patient; attach monitors; start peripheral IV and arterial line; sedation with midazolam; pulmonary artery catheter may be placed before induction
   B. Induction: rapid sequence; may use pentothal, ketamine, etomidate; succinylcholine and/or vecuronium or pancuronium bromide
   C. Maintenance: O_2-air-fentanyl citrate-isoflurane-relaxant
   D. Placement of lines: internal jugular introducers, left arm 9F introducer
   E. Padding of patient: arms, heels, sacrum
II. Stage I, Hepatectomy
   A. Goal: maintain adequate filling pressures to maintain cardiac output and blood pressure

B. Problems
   1. Bleeding from atrioventricular shunts, adhesions from prior operations
   2. Hemodynamic changes (including arrhythmia) secondary to inferior vena cava (IVC) manipulation, decreased venous return, and compression of pericardium by suprahepatic retraction
   3. Urine output
      a. Maintenance is crucial for prevention of acute tubular necrosis
      b. Infuse dopamine 2.5 μg/kg/min
      c. Manipulate with volume, furosemide, mannitol, dopamine based on filling pressures, electrolytes
   4. Hypoxemia is treated with high F_{IO_2}, PEEP
   5. Hypothermia
      a. Can increase systemic vascular resistance (SVR), cardiac irritability, myocardial depression and decrease GFR, hepatic blood flow, and hemoglobin P_{50}
      b. Accept 34°C as minimum temperature
      c. Temperature less than 32°C may affect coagulation
      d. Prevent with warm room, warming blanket, warmed IV fluids, humidifier (set at 38°–40°C)
   6. Hyperkalemia
      a. Correct with diuresis and replacement with fluid that does not contain K^+
      b. Treat with Ca^{++}, $D_{50}W$ plus insulin, sodium bicarbonate
   7. Hypocalcemia: $CaCl_2$ (1 g) needed to maintain CO and blood pressure when ionized Ca^{++} is below 1.2 mEq/L
   8. Anemia: maintain hematocrit 25%–32%
   9. Coagulation Defects
      a. One-third have essentially normal hemostasis throughout; one-third have bleeding diathesis during anhepatic phase; one-third have bleeding throughout
      b. Document factor deficiency and replace with appropriate products: fresh frozen plasma (FFP), platelets, cryoprecipitate, use thromboelastogram
         1. Prolonged R (reaction time): treat with FFP (2 Units) initially
         2. Decreased maximum amplitude (MA < 40 mm): treat with platelets (10 Units); narrow α angle: also treat with platelets

        3. Cryoprecipitate that contains fibrinogen, factor VIII, and factor XIII is given when FFP and platelets do not improve coagulation or when clot formation is slow ($\alpha < 45°$)

        4. Platelets, cryoprecipitate, and aminocaproic acid are withheld during veno-venous bypass to lessen risk of thromboembolism

  10. Porto-femoral-axillary vein bypass (veno-venous bypass)

      a. Embolism from lines

      b. Acute rise in central venous pressure (CVP), pulmonary artery pressure (PAP) secondary to increased superior vena cava flow

      c. Flow rate of 1–4 L/min desirable

      d. Transient hypothermia due to priming solution may cause bradycardia

III. Stage II, Anhepatic Phase

  A. Begins with hepatectomy and ends when vascular anastomoses of IVC and portal vein are complete; hepatic artery anastomosis can wait

  B. Problems

      1. Adverse hemodynamic changes secondary to decreased venous return are greatly modified by veno-venous bypass; as portal vein anastomosis is being done, partial bypass from femoral vein to left arm occurs with flows of 1–1.5 L/min

      2. Acidosis

          a. Patients with postoperative metabolic acidosis have high mortality; metabolic alkalosis is the rule due to citrate metabolism

          b. Treat with $NaHCO_3$ for base deficit greater than -5 mEq/L; excess $NaHCO_3$ may cause hypernatremia and hyperosmolality and may aggravate postoperative metabolic acidosis

      3. Hypocalcemia

          a. Follow Ca^{++}, QT interval, blood pressure, CVP

          b. Treat if $Ca^{++} < 1.2$ mEq/L

      4. Potassium abnormalities

          a. Mild hypokalemia is desirable in anticipation of K^+s efflux as donor liver is reperfused

          b. Treat hyperkalemia: $D_{50}W$ plus insulin in stage I

      5. Hypothermia

      6. Anemia

7. Coagulation abnormalities
8. Air embolism from veno-venous bypass or roller pump
9. Hydration: avoid fluid overload and pulmonary edema due to excessive crystalloid administration; try to keep pulmonary capillary wedge pressure on "dry side" during this phase, as increased PAP is seen after reperfusion; this procedure also allows "room" for blood left in bypass pump to be reinfused

C. Administer hydrocortisone 1 g IV before reperfusion

IV. Stage III, Reperfusion

    A. Begins with reperfusion of grafted liver by release of clamps on infrahepatic and suprahepatic vena cava and portal vein; sequence of clamp removal: infrahepatic-IVC, suprahepatic-IVC, portal vein

    B. Preparation

        1. Donor liver will be flushed with 250–500 mL of cold lactated Ringer's solution before reperfusion; flush via portal vein, exits liver from incomplete infrahepatic-IVC anastomosis

        2. Hydrocortisone 1 g IV before reperfusion

        3. Pretreat with $NaHCO_3$ 50–100 mEq and $CaCl_2$ 1 g about 1 minute before reperfusion to counteract hyperpotassemia

    C. Postreperfusion syndrome

        1. Hypotension, bradycardia, variable CO, ↑↑CVP, ↑↑PAP, ↓↓SVR; cannot accurately measure CO for about 5 minutes after reperfusion because of temperature changes

        2. Cardiovascular collapse: septal wall motion abnormalities

        3. Treat if necessary with atropine and/or epinephrine (5–10 μg boluses)

        4. Hyperkalemia: treat with $NaHCO_3$, $CaCl_2$, $D_{50}W$ plus insulin, as indicated

        5. Acidosis: treat with $NaHCO_3$ as indicated

        6. Hypothermia: core temperature may decrease 1°C with reperfusion; as donor liver begins to function, temperature will rise (as will CO_2 production and $ETCO_2$)

        7. Air embolism

        8. Cardiac arrest

        9. Coagulation

            a. Heparin effect: protamine may be indicated. Document with thromboelastogram using blood sample with protamine added (0.33 mL blood plus 0.03 mL protamine)

      b. Usually improves after 30–90 minutes if liver is functional

      c. Fibrinolysis possible; document with thromboelastogram before epsilon amino caproic acid 1 g, as this drug may cause thrombosis

    10. High CVP may cause congestion of liver; may need nitroglycerin, furosemide to decrease CVP; keep below 15 mm Hg, ideally 10–12 mm Hg

  D. Hepatic artery anastomosis

V. Stage IV, Neohepatic or Biliary Reconstruction

  A. Biliary reconstruction

    1. Duct-to-duct anastomosis (choledochocholedochostomy)

    2. Choledochojejunostomy to Roux-en-Y limb if inadequate biliary drainage caused by biliary atresia, biliary cirrhosis, or sclerosing cholangitis

  B. Post-transplantation problems

    1. Coagulation defects

    2. Hypothermia

    3. Surgical hemostasis

    4. Discontinuation of veno-venous bypass

    5. Closure; may be difficult secondary to distended and edematous bowel

References

1 Adler M, Gavaler JS, Duquesnoy R et al: Relationship between diagnosis, preoperative evaluation, and prognosis after orthotopic liver transplantation. Ann Surg 208:197, 1988

2. Rappaport AM, Borowy ZJ, Lougheed WM, Lotto WN: Subdivision of hexagonal liver lobules into a structural and functional unit. Anat Rec 119:16, 1954

3. Witte CL, Witte MH: Splanchnic circulatory and tissue fluid dynamics in portal hypertension. Federation Proceedings 42:1685, 1983

4. Vorobioff J, Bredfeldt JE, Groszmann RJ: Increased bloodflow through the portal system in cirrhotic rats. Gastroenterology 87:1120, 1984

5. Kretz R: Lebercirrhose. Patho Gesselch 8:54, 1904

6. Benoit JN, Womack WA, Hernandez L, Granger DN: "Forward" and "backward" flow mechanisms of portal hypertension. Gastroenterology 89:1092, 1985

7. Sherwin R, Joshi P, Hendler R, Felig P, Conn HO: Hyperglucagonemia in Laennec's cirrhosis: The role of porta-systemic shunting. N Engl J Med 290:239, 1974

8. Benoit JN, Barrowman JA, Harper SL, Kvietys PR, Granger DN: Role of humoral factors in the intestinal hyperemia associated with chronic portal hypertension. Am J Physiol 247:G486, 1984

9. Julik TJ, Johnson DE, Elde RP, Lock JE: Pulmonary vascular effects of vaso-active intestinal peptide in conscious newborn lambs. Am J Physiol 246:H716, 1984

10. Keren G, Boichis H, Zwas TS, Frand M: Pulmonary arterio-venous fistulae in hepatic cirrhosis. Arch Dis Child 58:302, 1983

11. Henriksen JH, Christensen NJ, Ring-Larsen J: Noradrenaline and adrenaline in various vascular beds in patients with cirrhosis: Relation to haemodynamics. Clin Physiol 1:293, 1981

12. Kiel JW, Pitts V, Benoit JN, Granger DN, Shepherd AP: Reduced vascular sensitivity to norepinephrine in portal-hypertensive rats. Am J Physiol 248:G192, 1985

13. Richardson PDI, Withrington PG: Glucagon inhibition of hepatic arterial responses to hepatic nerve stimulation. Am J Physiol 233:H647, 1977

14. Bosch J, Arroyo V, Betriu A et al: Hepatic hemodynamics and the renin-angiotensin-aldosterone system in cirrhosis. Gastroenterology 78:92, 1980

15. Epstein M: Renal functional abnormalities in cirrhosis: Pathophysiology and management. In Zakim D, Boyer TD (eds): Hepatology: A Textbook of Liver Disease, p. 446. Philadelphia, WB Saunders, 1982

16. Perez-Ayuso RM, Arroyo V, Camps J et al: Renal kallikrein excretion in cirrhotics with ascites: Relationship to renal hemodynamics. Hepatology 4:247, 1984

17. Racz K, Buu NT, Kucel O, DeLean A: Dopamine 3-sulfate inhibits aldosterone secretion in cultured bovine adrenal cells. Am J Physiol 247:E431, 1984

18. Gazzard BG, Rake MO, Flute PT et al: Bleeding in relation to the coagulation defect of fulminant hepatic failure. In Williams R, Murray-Lyon IM (eds): Artificial Liver Support, p. 63. Tunbridge Wells, England, Pitman Medical, 1975

19. Dymock IW, Tucker JS, Woolf IL et al: Coagulation studies as a prognostic index in acute liver failure. Br J Haematol 29:385, 1975

20. Flute PT: Blood coagulation defects in FHF. Am J Gastroenterol 69:363, 1978

21. Verstraete M, Vermylen J, Collen D: Intravascular coagulation in liver disease. Ann Rev Med 25:447, 1974

22. B'oom AL: Intravascular coagulation and the liver. Br J Haematol 30:1, 1975

23. Van Theil DH, Tarter R, Stone BG: Pathophysiology of liver disease in hepatic transplantation. In Winter PM, Kang YG (eds): Hepatic Transplantation: Anesthetic and Perioperative Management, p. 31. New York, Praeger, 1986

24. Shelly MP, Park G, Powell-Jackson P: Morphine in patients following liver transplantation. Presented at the 4th World Congress on Intensive and Critical Care Medicine, Jerusalem, June 1985

25. Laidlaw J, Read AE, Sherlock S: Morphine tolerance in hepatic cirhosis. Gastroenterology 40;389, 1961

26. Branch RA, Morgan MH, James J et al: Intravenous administration of diazepam in patients with chronic liver disease. Gut 17:975, 1976

27. MacGilchrist AJ, Birnie GC, Cook A et al: Pharmacokinetics and pharmacodynamics of intravenous midazolam in patients with severe alcoholic cirrhosis. Gut 27:190, 1986

28. Pandele G, Chaux F, Salvadori C et al: Thiopental pharmacokinetics in patients with cirrhosis. Anesthesiology 59:123, 1983
29. Kang YG, Uram M, Shin GK et al: The pharmacokinetics of fentanyl and end-stage liver disease. Anesthesiology 61:A380, 1984
30. Ferrier C, Marty J, Bouffard Y et al: Alfentanil pharmacokinetics in patients with cirrhosis. Anesthesiology 62:480, 1985
31. Baraka A, Bagali F: Correlation between tubocurarine requirements and plasma protein pattern. Br J Anaesth 40:89, 1968
32. Arden JR, Lynam DP, Castagnoli KP et al: Vecuronium and alcoholic liver disease: Pharmacokinetic and pharmacodynamic analysis. Anesthesiology 68:771, 1988
33. Ward S, Neill AM: Pharmacokinetics of atracurium in acute hepatic failure. Br J Anaesth 55:1169, 1983
34. Green AJ, Ratnoff OD: Elevated antihemophilic factor (AHF, factor VIII) procoagulant activity and AHF-like antigen in alcoholic cirrhosis of the liver. J Lab Clin Med 83:189, 1974
35. Karpatkin S, Freedman ML. Hypersplenic thrombocytopenia differentiated from increased peripheral destruction by platelet volume. Ann Intern Med 89:200, 1978
36. Bontempo FA, Lewis JH, Ragni MV et al: The preoperative coagulation pattern in liver transplant patients. In Winter PM, Kang YG (eds): Hepatic Transplantation: Anesthetic and Perioperative Management. New York, Praeger, 1986
37. Kang YG, Martin DJ, Marquez J et al: Intraoperative changes in blood coagulation and thromboelastographic monitoring in liver transplantation. Anesth Analg 64:888, 1985
38. Kang YG: Monitoring and treatment of coagulation. In Winter PM, Kang YG (eds): Hepatic Transplantation: Anesthetic and Perioperative Management. New York, Praeger, 1986
39. Munson ES, Merrick HC: Effects of nitrous oxide on venous embolism. Anesthesiology 27:783, 1966
40. Nagano K, Gelman S, Parks D, Bradley E: Hepatic oxygen supply-uptake relationship and metabolism during anesthesia in miniature pigs. Anesthesiology 72:902, 1990
41. Nagano K, Gelman S, Parks D, Bradley EL: Hepatic circulation and oxygen supply-uptake relationships after hepatic ischemic insult during anesthesia with volatile anesthetics and fentanyl in miniature pigs. Anesth Analg 70:53, 1990
42. Winter PM, Kang YG: Hepatic Transplantation: Anesthetic and Perioperative Management. New York, Praeger, 1986

Verdi J. DiSesa

Immunosuppression for Cardiac
8 Transplantation

The first successful organ transplants were performed in 1954. The recipients of these kidney grafts did not receive immunosuppression. These organ transplantations were successful, however, because the donor was the twin of the recipient and therefore genetically identical. For this reason, the organ graft caused no immune response. Subsequent organ transplants between nonidentical relatives or nonrelated individuals required the development of immunosuppressive drugs that would temper the body's immune response to foreign tissue. Immune suppression, therefore, has made present day organ transplantation possible.

While immune suppression is necessary for organ transplantation, however, most of the ills and complications suffered by organ transplant recipients are related to either the primary or side effects of immunosuppressive drugs. Most patients live in a state of partial tolerance to their transplanted organ. Levels of immunosuppression adequate to totally suppress the immune response would leave a patient liable to life-threatening infection. Patients therefore remain suspended between inadequate immunosuppression and life-threatening or at least graft-threatening rejection, and over-immunosuppression and life-threatening infection. In addition, the drugs commonly used today have significant secondary side effects, including nephrotoxicity, hepatotoxicity, neurotoxicity, alteration of body habitus, glucose intolerance, and personality changes.

This chapter discusses current immunosuppression in organ transplantation, using cardiac transplantation as a paradigm. Most of the drugs used in organ transplantations are used in cardiac transplantation and most of the issues are the same. One advantage that the physician who cares for the heart transplant recipient has is that fairly clear-cut definitions of rejection are available based on histologic analysis of endomyocardial biopsy. Therefore, reliance need not be placed on secondary functional assays of organ viability, such as serum creatinine in renal transplantation or serum glucose in pancreatic transplantation. Heart transplantation is different in other ways. Unlike kidney transplantation, histocompatibility matching is not done before heart transplantation, and, of course, living related heart donation is not a possibility. However, these facts do not mean that histocompatibility matching does not have an impact on the results of heart transplantation. Both single-center studies and a large multi-institutional study appear to show the beneficial impact of fortuitous tissue matching on the results of heart transplantation.[1,2] Patients who share one or more HLA-A, -B, or -DR tissue antigens appear to have improved graft survival, just as in kidney transplantation. At present, however, prospective tissue matching is not possible in cardiac transplantation.

This review therefore focuses on strategies of immunosuppression and the immunosuppressive agents used to treat the recipients of heart transplantation who have not had prospective histocompatibility tissue matching. Immunosuppression for heart transplantation has evolved in parallel with the development of drugs and techniques in other organ transplantation. Presently, the consensus is that immunosuppression with triple drug therapy (i.e., prednisone, cyclosporine, and azathioprine) is the standard in heart transplantation.[3,4]

As has been suggested by others, three distinct phases of immunosuppression occur in heart transplantation.[5] These include the induction or prophylactic phase, the maintenance phase, and treatment of acute

TABLE 8-1. A Typical
Immunoprophylactic Regimen

Agent	Dosage Schedule
OKT3	Days 0–14
Cyclosporine	Start day 7
Corticosteroids	Start day 0
Azathioprine	Start day 0

rejection episodes. This review considers immunosuppression from the perspective of each of these distinct phases in the immune management of the heart transplant recipient. In addition, it includes a discussion of the mechanisms of action of these agents, as well as the significant complications that they may cause. Finally, the review concludes with a discussion of some new concepts in immunosuppression.

INDUCTION THERAPY: EARLY REJECTION PROPHYLAXIS

Induction, or prophylactic immunosuppression, is based on an intense period of early immunosuppression after engraftment (Table 8-1). Theoretically, early and intense immune therapy, by eliminating effector cells important in the early recognition phase of the immune response, might enhance long-term graft tolerance. Most induction regimens in heart transplantation use either polyclonal (antithymocyte globulin [ATG] or antilymphocyte globulin [ALG]) or monoclonal (OKT3) anti-lymphocyte antibodies.[6-13] These agents attack either all lymphocytes or specifically T lymphocytes thought to be important initiators in graft rejection. When used early, these agents have been shown to delay the onset of the first rejection episode. This delay constitutes another rationale for use of induction or prophylactic therapy.

Patients are usually most unstable from a hemodynamic, nutritional, and constitutional point of view in the early days after heart transplantation. By definition, all heart transplant recipients have end-stage heart failure, and many have latent or incipient dysfunction of other organs because of heart failure. Therefore, the rationale is to delay rejection, which may cause further hemodynamic instability, until the patient has recovered from the insult of surgery and the underlying problems of chronic heart failure. In addition, the newly transplanted heart has suffered an ischemic injury that may make it more susceptible to the deleterious hemodynamic effects of acute rejection.

Finally, induction therapy has been proposed as a method to limit the toxicity of the other agents used for maintenance immunosuppression, particularly cyclosporine.[14] One of the chief toxicities of cyclosporine is impairment of renal function. Patients with heart failure may already have compromised renal function at the time of transplantation and in the early days after surgery. While this dysfunction occurs usually on the basis of low cardiac output, it may be exacerbated by time spent on cardiopulmonary bypass. In some immunosuppressive protocols, cyclosporine therapy is not begun until several days after transplantation, at which time the kidneys have had a chance to recover. To maintain adequate levels of immunosuppression in these early days, prophylactic therapy with ATG or OKT3 has been proposed.

As noted, the agents usually used for induction or prophylactic therapy include ATG, ALG, or the mouse monoclonal antibody OKT3. The polyclonal antibodies ATG and ALG are made by immunizing animals with thymocytes or lymphocytes. Serum of the immunized animals is then collected and administered, usually over a 7- to 14-day interval. Obviously, the specificity and potency of an individual batch of ATG or ALG may be variable. In addition, the dose is necessarily arbitrary and empiric. However, a large amount of experience with these agents has accrued over the years, and their administration has become relatively standardized. The OKT3 is a monoclonal mouse antibody to an antigen present on all T cells. It is made from single clones of immunoglobulin-producing cells using modern techniques of molecular biology. It is, therefore, standardized and its effects more reproducible. These properties give it a theoretic advantage over the other agents.

Numerous studies have been performed to evaluate the efficacy of induction or prophylactic therapy using these agents. A number of regimens have been tried. In most cases, a short course of induction therapy with one of these agents has been combined with standard triple immunosuppression with cyclosporine, prednisone, and azathioprine. Several studies from the University of Pittsburgh have purported to show an advantage when ATG prophylaxis was used.[9],[11,13] This group has seen a significantly higher incidence of rejection in the first 30 days in patients who received OKT3 as compared to those who received ATG. For example, by the end of the first month after transplantation, 25% of patients who received ATG had experienced a rejection episode compared with nearly 50% of those who received OKT3. These investigators observed this difference as long as 4 months after transplantation. In addition, the incidence of second episodes of rejection was higher in the group that received OKT3 prophylaxis (50%) as compared to the group that received ATG (35%).

Investigators from Pittsburgh also observed significantly more lymphocyte growth from endomyocardial biopsies in patients treated with OKT3 as opposed to ATG.[12] They also saw significantly greater donor-specific cytotoxic activity in the biopsy-grown cultures of the OKT3-treated patients. They concluded that ATG therapy reduced the incidence of cellular rejection as compared with OKT3 immunoprophylaxis.

Other studies, however, have suggested that OKT3 is as effective as other forms of immunoprophylaxis.[5,7] Studies from the University of Utah showed that OKT3 was more effective in decreasing the risk of early rejection when compared to an ATG-based protocol.[5] In addition, the Utah group was able to discontinue maintenance steroids more frequently in patients treated prophylactically with OKT3. This fact was associated with a decreased propensity to late rejection in the OKT3-treated group. In contrast, studies from the University of Alabama have failed to show a difference between polyclonal ATG and monoclonal OKT3 given as prophylactic induction therapy.[6]

As noted, one rationale for induction therapy has been to limit the early toxicity of cyclosporine and other agents. Emery and associates used induction immunosuppression in patients bridged to transplantation with mechanical devices.[14] Obviously, these patients are among the most compromised patients referred for transplantation. These investigators used an immunosuppressive regimen based on immunoprophylaxis with OKT3. They were able to modify the doses of other immunosuppressives and, in several of their patients, ultimately to eliminate maintenance steroids. They observed a low overall incidence of rejection (0.22 episodes per patient) and, on this basis, have expanded their indications for a modified regimen using OKT3. They have applied this type of immunosuppression in patients with preoperative organ dysfunction, in diabetic patients, and in those who require mechanical assistance after transplantation.

Despite these favorable studies, a consensus in favor of immunoprophylaxis with some form of antilymphocyte antibody does not exist. While there is widespread agreement that immunoprophylaxis can delay the onset of the first rejection episode, the overall incidence of rejection may not be appreciably changed by this form of therapy.[15] More important is the fact that a significant incidence of complications is related to early, intense immunosuppression. Increased rates of infection have been observed in patients treated with immunoprophylactic regimens.[16] In addition, the agents themselves, particularly OKT3, may cause significant febrile and adverse hemodynamic reactions when they are first administered. These may not be tolerated well in the heart transplant patient early after operation. Finally, all of these antibody preparations are made in nonhuman mammals; therefore, the recipient could possibly develop antibodies to the foreign proteins. Theoretically, at least, these antibodies may limit the effectiveness of subsequent doses of these agents. As these are the primary agents used as rescue therapy for persistent or intractable rejection, there is a theoretic disadvantage to using them early and thereby potentially limiting their subsequent effectiveness. For all of these reasons, induction regimens are only used in about half of the transplant programs in this country. This fact may change as further data based on refinements in therapy become available.

CHRONIC MAINTENANCE IMMUNOSUPPRESSION

The introduction of cyclosporine in the early 1980s appeared to trigger a revolution in the management of patients after heart transplantation. The use of cyclosporine was associated with a dramatic improvement in the results of heart transplantation and a corresponding dramatic increase in interest and application of heart transplantation. While the explosive growth in heart transplantation probably was due as much to improvements in the general care of these patients as to the introduction of cyclosporine, most immunosuppressive regimens today are built around the use of this agent. Maintenance immunosuppressive protocols are designed to prevent allograft rejection without the infectious side effects of over-immunosuppression. Most maintenance immunosuppressive protocols are based on combinations of prednisone, cyclosporine, and azathioprine (Table 8-2).[5] Some centers make a concerted effort to eliminate maintenance steroids and treat patients with cyclosporine and azathioprine alone, if possible.[5,17]

One poorly understood but reproducible observation is that higher doses of immunosuppression are required early after transplantation. Subsequently, doses of drugs, especially corticosteroids, can be reduced without necessarily triggering an acute rejection episode. A high dose of steroids, usually in the form of prednisone, is administered in the early days after a transplantation. Doses may be as high as 1000 mg or more on the first day but are usually tapered to about 30 mg per day in the

TABLE 8-2. Maintenance Immunosuppression

Agent	Dose	Comments
Cyclosporine	3–8 mg/kg/day	Blood level 150–250 ng/mL
Corticosteroids	0.5 mg/kg/day of prednisone equivalent	Taper to 0.1 mg/kg/day
Azathioprine	2–4 mg/kg/day	White blood cell count ≥ 5000/mm^3

adult patient 2 weeks after transplantation. In the ensuing weeks and months after transplantation, the dose of steroids is weaned so that, by 1 year, most patients are maintained on 2 to 5 mg of prednisone a day. As noted, in some centers steroids are eliminated completely as long as recurrent acute rejection does not ensue.

Cyclosporine dosage is titrated both to maintain a certain blood level and to avoid toxicity, which is predominantly renal and less often hepatic. Immediately postoperatively, patients may be maintained on a continuous infusion of cyclosporine (1 mg/kg/day). This regimen assures absorption and seems to minimize toxicity. Subsequently, the patient may be switched to an oral dose (3–8 mg/kg/day) when enteral intake resumes. In the early weeks after transplantation, cyclosporine levels are maintained at about 250 ng/mL. The dose is reduced if azotemia develops. With chronic cyclosporine administration, elevations in serum creatinine as high as 2 to 2.5 mg/dL are common. Usually, by 2 to 3 months after transplantation, the cyclosporine level can be reduced to 150 to 200 ng/mL, which usually allows for stable, although mildly impaired, renal function. One of the difficulties in caring for patients who are taking cyclosporine is the variability of absorption of this drug as well as the variability in the assays used to detect it in blood. A number of assays are available, and, while they are improving, adjustment of cyclosporine dosing remains an art.[18–22]

Doses of azathioprine are usually given at 1 to 2 mg/kg, as long as the white blood count remains above 5000/mm³. The dosage may be increased to two times this level or higher if a concerted effort is being made to eliminate maintenance corticosteroids. Again, adjustments in dosage are made if the white blood count drops below safe levels, generally 4000 to 5000/mm³.

In an effort to avoid the side effects of chronic steroid administration, including changes in body habitus, hypertension, wound healing difficulties, osteoporosis, and glucose intolerance, a number of centers have investigated corticosteroid-free maintenance immunosuppression.[5,17,23,24] In general, attempts have been made to wean corticosteroids completely by 6 weeks to 3 months after cardiac transplantation. Recurrent or persistent rejection is the usual reason for failure of these regimens and reinstitution of steroid therapy. Patients successfully weaned off steroids appear to have fewer problems with hypercholesterolemia, obesity, infection, and hypertension. At present, it is not possible to predict which patients will be successfully managed without steroids. Present results suggest that female patients can less often be managed without steroids, but the basis for this difference is poorly understood.

MECHANISMS OF ACTION OF
IMMUNOSUPPRESSIVE AGENTS

Corticosteroids are potent anti-inflammatory drugs. Inflammation and nonspecific cytodestructive mechanisms play a significant role in rejection, and corticosteroids have a role in combating these effects. Relatively convincing evidence shows that corticosteroids block the production of a number of inflammatory cytokines, including prostaglandins and leukotrienes.[25] The production of several important immune cytokines, such as interleukin-1 (IL-1) and tumor necrosis factor, appears to be significantly inhibited by corticosteroids. Steroids may also inhibit transcription of inflammatory mediators such as IL-6. The activity of IL-2 may also be affected by steroid administration. Both the transcription of IL-2 and its release may be blocked directly or indirectly by steroid administration.

Azathioprine is an antimetabolite that acts on the DNA synthetic (S) phase of the cellular cycle.[25] This drug belongs to the class of molecules called thiopurines. Its active component, 6-mercaptopurine, is produced by cleavage in the liver. 6-mercaptopurine was the first available immunosuppressive drug. This cytotoxic agent appears to have preferential action on T cells and thus has the potential to prevent proliferation of activated lymphocytes.

Cyclosporine, the product of a fungus, is a cyclic peptide. It is highly fat soluble and diffuses passively through cell membranes, where it binds to intracellular proteins. The molecular basis for its subsequent actions are poorly understood. However, evidence suggests that cyclosporine and a cytoplasmic protein (cyclophilin) form a complex that penetrates the nucleus and inhibits the production of messenger RNA in T cells.[25] Cyclophilin is an isomerase, a class of enzymes important in protein folding. How such an enzyme is related to the cellular effects of cyclosporine is unclear. Cyclosporine affects the production and action of IL-2 and almost certainly other mediators as well.

As noted, OKT3 is a mouse monoclonal antibody directed against an antigen on the surface of all T cells. The T cell receptor is associated with a complex of peptides known as CD3. The OKT3 antibody is directed to an epitope on one of the peptides that makes up the CD3 complex. OKT3 binds to CD3, which is present on all T cells, and leads most likely to complement-dependent lysis of the cells and possibly to lymphocyte opsonization. OKT3 may also produce inactivation of CD3 positive cells without lysis. The molecular basis for these effects is unknown.

The mechanisms of action of the polyclonal antilymphocyte and antithymocyte sera are not well understood. Presumably, these antibodies bind to a variety of epitopes present on lymphocytes, causing their destruction or inactivation. Measurable lymphopenia is demonstrable after treatment with all of the antilymphocyte antibody preparations and is further evidence that depletion of active immune cells is an important component of their mechanisms of action.

THE TREATMENT OF ACUTE REJECTION

In the cardiac allograft, rejection is diagnosed by the histologic appearance of endomyocardial biopsies.[5,26] In the cyclosporine era, the clinical manifestations of acute rejection may be subtle or absent. In episodes of severe rejection, hemodynamic compromise may occur; the goal of surveillance therapy, however, is to detect rejection before obvious functional deterioration occurs. In most patients treated with cyclosporine, some degree of lymphocyte infiltration is frequently present on biopsies. Lymphocyte infiltration in the absence of myocyte necrosis usually is not treated.[27] Moderate rejection, characterized by lymphocyte infiltration with myocyte necrosis, almost always requires treatment. Severe rejection with widespread infiltrates and necrosis and possible associated vasculitis and hemorrhage may require multimodality antirejection therapy and, as noted, may be accompanied by transient hemodynamic collapse.

The basic principle of all antirejection therapy is to administer a short course of intense immunosuppression (Table 8-3). The usual first therapy for moderate rejection is a pulse of steroids, given intravenously (IV) over a 3-day period.[28,29] Five hundred to 1000 mg of IV prednisolone are given daily for 3 days with follow-up biopsy performed 1 week to 10 days after completion of the pulse. In patients with milder forms of rejection, an oral pulse of prednisone may be substituted.[30] In some cases, short-term intensification of cyclosporine dosage may be effective for treatment of moderate rejection.

TABLE 8-3. Therapy of Acute Rejection

Rejection	Treatment
Moderate	Methyl prednisolone 1000 mg IV daily for 3 days
Severe or Persistent	Prednisolone plus either OKT3 5 mg IV daily for 10 days *or* ALG 20 mg/kg IV daily for 10–14 days

Severe rejection or moderate rejection that does not respond to one or two steroid pulses usually is treated with an antilymphocyte antibody. No advantage to ATG, ALG, or OKT3 can be demonstrated, and the agent used often depends on availability at a particular center. Occasionally, a rejection episode that does not respond to one antilymphocyte antibody may respond to another. Therefore, patients who fail a course of ATG may respond to OKT3 or ALG, and vice versa. The production of antimouse antibodies may limit the effectiveness of subsequent doses of OKT3. Antibody levels are usually checked after a course of OKT3. However, despite this theoretic possibility, multiple courses of OKT3 can be given if clinically indicated. If antimouse antibody levels are detected, a higher dose of OKT3 may be necessary. Levels of circulating CD3- positive lymphocytes are followed during the course of OKT3 therapy. Although the relationship between CD3-positive cell levels and response to rejection has not been established, the dose of OKT3 may be increased if levels do not fall significantly.

In most cases, these protocols lead to successful resolution of rejection. In one study, 85% of initial episodes of acute allograft rejection responded to a course of IV corticosteroids.[29] A recent study has addressed the issue of whether doses as high as 1 g of prednisone per day are required in a steroid pulse.[31] These investigators compared the standard 1 g/day regimens to 500 mg and 250 mg/day courses of treatment. These authors observed comparable resolution of rejection in all three groups, despite marked reduction in the total dose of steroids. In the setting of triple-drug immunosuppression, these authors felt that the lower dose steroids might reduce side effects without jeopardizing the response to rejection.

Another recent study compared treatment of refractory rejection with OKT3 to that using ALG.[32] These authors found that a significantly larger number of patients responded to the first course of OKT3, but that, after repeat therapy with ALG, resolution of rejection was the same in both groups. In this study, a significantly increased incidence of infection was observed in patients treated with OKT3, and on this basis ALG was the recommended therapy for refractory rejection.

While these studies suggest that some modifications or refinements in antirejection therapy may be available by subtle adjustments in standard protocols, results differ little. The standard of therapy of rejection remains initial treatment with a short pulse of corticosteroids, accompanied by some form of ALG if rejection is severe or if hemodynamics are compromised. Refractory episodes of rejection are treated with OKT3 or one of the polyclonal globulin formulations.

COMPLICATIONS OF IMMUNOSUPPRESSIVE THERAPY

All of the agents used for maintenance immune suppression have significant side effects (Table 8-4).[33,34] As previously mentioned, glucocorticoids cause glucose intolerance, lead to increased body mass, and produce osteoporosis. These are not trivial side effects. Not only can they decrease patient satisfaction with the outcome of transplantation, but they can predispose to infection and problems with wound healing. Patients who take steroids are susceptible to bone destruction and orthopedic injuries that require corrective surgery. Major morbidity may result from vertebral osteoporosis and compression fractures of the spine, which are difficult to treat and cause significant disability. Glucocorticoids may also contribute to hypertension and hyperlipidemia.[35] While these agents have not been implicated directly in the development of graft coronary atherosclerosis, hypertension and hyperlipidemia probably contribute to this process.

Cyclosporine has significant side effects, the most obvious of which is nephrotoxicity.[36-39] Almost all patients maintained on chronic cyclosporine have elevations in serum creatinine to 2 mg/dL or higher. Generalized sympathetic hyper-reactivity has been detected in patients who are receiving cyclosporine and may be responsible for the abnormalities

TABLE 8-4.   Side Effects of Immunosuppressive Agents

Agent	Side Effects
Cyclosporine	Hepatotoxicity
	Hirsutism
	Hypertension
	Nephrotoxicity
	Seizures
Corticosteroids	Changes in body habitus
	Glucose intolerance
	Hyperlipidemia
	Hypertension
	Obesity
	Osteoporosis
	Personality changes
Azathioprine	Anemia
	Hepatotoxicity
	Leukopenia
	Thrombocytopenia

in renal function. Sympathetic hyper-reactivity also may be the cause of the hypertension that is observed in almost all patients treated with cyclosporine.[40-42] Cyclosporine may contribute to hypertension by its nephrotoxic effects as well.

Cyclosporine is also hepatotoxic. Hepatocellular toxicity usually responds to a decrease in the dosage. Cyclosporine may produce significant cholestasis.[43] While cyclosporine has not been implicated in the development of gallstones, if present they should be treated aggressively, as acute cholecystitis may not be tolerated well in the immunosuppressed patient. Cyclosporine may also lower the seizure threshold and predispose patients with previous neurologic insults to further difficulties. Finally, cyclosporine may significantly interact with the absorption of other fat-soluble medications; therefore, care must be taken in the institution or withdrawal of other pharmacologic therapy.

Azathioprine has predominant hematologic toxicity as well as hepatotoxicity. As noted, careful monitoring of white blood cell counts is part of standard therapy for patients maintained on this drug. Other hematologic abnormalities such as anemia and thrombocytopenia may also be secondary to azathioprine therapy. This toxicity should be suspected if these other abnormalities occur.

Immunosuppressed patients are also subject to a number of nonspecific complications. There is a fairly high incidence of abdominal catastrophes, including acute cholecystitis and perforated viscera in patients immunosuppressed after heart transplantation.[44,45] The etiology of these complications is not always clear. It is most likely a combination of the side effects of immunosuppressive drugs, the stresses of chronic heart failure magnified by the acute stresses of the heart transplant operation and cardiopulmonary bypass, and underlying atherosclerotic cardiovascular disease, which affects a significant number of transplant patients. Patients managed with cyclosporine and azathioprine may also be susceptible to the development of malignancies that are most often lymphoproliferative in nature.[46] Fortunately, many of these respond to reduction in drug dosage. However, the reductions in medication that are usually required often predispose the patient to life-threatening episodes of rejection.

NEW CONCEPTS IN IMMUNOSUPPRESSION FOR HEART TRANSPLANTATION

As this discussion has emphasized, present-day immunosuppression is far from perfect. The incomplete, nonspecific suppression of the immune response to the grafted tissues leaves the patient vulnerable to rejection and infection as well as the nonimmunologic side effects of the agents used. Research on new agents for immunosuppression and new concepts of immunosuppression is, for obvious reasons, one of the most active areas in transplant research.

A number of adjunctive agents have been tried in order to enhance immunosuppression while minimizing side effects. Vincristine sulfate has been used as an additive agent to standard immunosuppression in heart transplantation.[47] In a prospective trial performed at the University of Utah, vincristine sulfate was given after OKT3 induction. While no significant differences in survival, infection, or amounts of other immunosuppressive agents used were found, the patients with higher risk for rejection appeared to do better when vincristine was added to their immunosuppressive regimen. Neuropathy was a major side effect that occurred in nearly half of the patients, however.

Bromocriptine has been used as an adjuvant to cyclosporine immunosuppression in heart transplantation.[48] Bromocriptine inhibits the pituitary release of prolactin, which apparently competes with cyclosporine for receptors on lymphocytes. In a prospective trial, bromocriptine improved the immunosuppressive effect of cyclosporine, especially during the early postoperative period. These investigators saw significantly higher freedom from infection and rejection, especially during the first 2 months after heart transplantation.

In some patients, rejection is persistent despite treatment with all known pharmacologic immunotherapy. In certain individuals, a course of total lymphoidal radiation has been effective for otherwise refractory rejection episodes.[49] This modality has not found a standard place in the management of heart transplant patients but may be a useful adjunct to future protocols.[50]

A number of experimental agents have been tried in heart transplantation, both in the laboratory and the clinic. FK506, a fungal product like cyclosporine, is among the better known of these agents.[51] It has been studied in a relatively small number of centers but apparently with good results in a variety of organ transplant settings. Nephrotoxicity has occurred in patients who received this drug, but, unlike cyclosporine, significant hypertension has not been observed. Whether it will be an improvement over cyclosporine is not yet clear. Other agents such as deoxysperguilan have been tried in experimental animal models but at present have no clinical role.[52]

A number of other approaches based on a more sophisticated understanding of the molecular biology of the immune response may one day have a significant place in the management of heart and other organ transplant recipients.[53] Monoclonal antibodies to lymphocyte activation antigens, such as the receptor for IL-2, are presently under investigation. Antibodies to CD4, an antigen present on T helper cells, have been investigated. Recipient pretreatment with combinations of prospective donor antigen and anti-CD4 have yielded promising results in experimental animals.

Other novel approaches to graft-specific immunosuppression have included manipulation of the thymic environment of the allograft recipient.[54] These techniques have significant theoretic appeal, since it is within the thymus that the education of lymphocytes takes place. The ultimate goal of transplant biology is to re-educate the immune system to recognize and accept the graft tissue as self. These preliminary investigations in thymic manipulations are promising initiatives in the induction of antigen-specific tolerance.

CONCLUSION

This review has explored present-day principles of immunosuppression for heart transplantation as a paradigm for immunosuppression for all organ transplantation. The major achievements of modern-day immunosuppression have been emphasized, along with the major limitations and complications of immune therapy. Areas of active investigation and new modalities of treatment for organ transplant recipients have been discussed. This is an exciting area of transplant biology that, when combined with the deeper understanding of the immune system that modern molecular biology is providing, will lead to significant advances in the care of these patients in the future.

References

1. DiSesa VJ, Kuo PC, Horvath KA, Mudge GH, Collins JJ Jr, Cohn LH: HLA histocompatibility affects cardiac transplant rejection and may provide one basis for organ allocation. Ann Thorac Surg 49:220, 1990
2. Opelz G: Effect of HLA matching in heart transplantation: Collaborative heart transplant study. Transplant Proc 21:794, 1989
3. Woodley SL, Renlund DG, O'Connell JB, Bristow MR: Immunosuppression following cardiac transplantation. Cardiol Clin 8:83, 1990
4. Casale AS, Reitz BA, Greene PS, Augustine S, Baumgartner WA: Immunosuppression after heart transplantation: Prednisone and cyclosporine with and without azathioprine. J Thorac Cardiovasc Surg 98:951, 1989
5. Renlund DG, O'Connell JB, Bristow MR: Strategies of immunosuppression in cardiac transplantation. Seminars in Thoracic and Cardiovascular Surgery 2:181, 1990
6. Kirklin JK, Bourge RC, White WD et al: Prophylactic therapy for rejection

after cardiac transplantation: A comparison of rabbit antithymocyte globulin and OKT3. J Thorac Cardiovasc Surg 99:716, 1990

7. Starnes VA, Oyer PE, Stinson EB, Dein JR, Shumway NE: Prophylactic OKT3 used as induction therapy for heart transplantation. Circulation 80:79, 1989

8. Copeland JG, Ocenogle TB, Williams RJ et al: Rabbit antithymocyte globulin: A 10-year experience in cardiac transplantation. J Thorac Cardiovasc Surg 99:852, 1990

9. Griffith BP, Kormos RL, Armitage JM, Dummer JS, Hardesty RL: Comparative trial of immunoprophylaxis with RATG versus OKT3. 9:301, 1990

10. Carey JA, Frist WH: Use of polyclonal antilymphocytic preparations for prophylaxis in heart transplantation. J Heart Transplant 9:297, 1990

11. Kormos RL, Herlan DB, Armitage JM et al: Monoclonal versus polyclonal antibody therapy for prophylaxis against rejection after heart transplantation. J Heart Transplant 9:1, 1990

12. Kaufman C, Zeevi A, Zerbe T et al: In vitro studies of endomyocardial biopsies from heart transplant recipients on RATG and OKT3 immunoprophylaxis protocols. Transplantation 48:621, 1989

13. Kormos RL, Armitage JM, Dummer JS, Miyamoto Y, Griffith BP, Hardesty RL: Optimal perioperative immunosuppression in cardiac transplantation using rabbit antithymocyte globulin. Transplantation 49:306, 1990

14. Emery RW, Joyce LD, Pritzker MR: Induction immunosuppression for patients bridged to transplantation. J Heart Transplant 9:316, 1990

15. Kobashigawa J, Stevenson LW, Moriguchi J et al: A randomized trial of short course OKT3 induction versus initial triple therapy: Impact on rejection and renal function after cardiac transplantation (abstr). J Am Coll Cardiol 10:163, 1991

16. Constanzo NMR, O'Sullivan EJ, Johnson MR et al: Prospective randomized trial of OKT3 versus horse antithymocyte globulin-based immunosuppressive prophylaxis in heart transplantation. J Heart Transplant 9:306, 1990

17. Laufer G, Laczkovics A, Wollenek G, Schreiner W, Wolner E: Results of orthotopic heart transplantation with and without the use of maintenance steroids. European Journal of Cardiothoracic Surgery 2:237, 1988

18. Zucchelli GC, Clerico A, Pilo A et al: Evaluation and comparison of radioimmunoassay methods using monoclonal or polyclonal antibodies for the assay of cyclosporine in blood samples. Int J Tissue React 11:315, 1989

19. Keown PA, Glenn J, Denegri J et al: Therapeutic monitoring of cyclosporine: Impact of a change in standards on 125I-monoclonal RIA performance in comparison with liquid chromatography. Clin Chem 36:804, 1990

20. Rondanelli R, Ragazzi MB, Gastaldi L, Legnazzi P, Abelli P: Measurement of cyclosporine in plasma of cardiac allograft recipients by fluorescence polarization immunoassay. Ther Drug Monit 12:182, 1990

21. Zylber-Katz E, Granit L: Cyclosporine blood concentrations determined by different assay methods in heart transplant patients. Ther Drug Monit 11:592, 1989

22. Hirvisalo EL, Kivisto KT, Neuvonen PJ: Therapeutic cyclosporine monitoring: Comparison of radioimmunoassay and high-performance liquid chromatography methods in organ transplant recipients. Ther Drug Monit 12:353, 1990

23. Ratkovec RM, Wray RB, Renlund DG et al: Influence of corticosteroid-free

maintenance of immunosuppression on allograft coronary artery disease after cardiac transplantation. J Thorac Cardiovasc Surg 100:6, 1990

24. Gorensek MJ, Stewart RW, Keys TF et al: Decreased infections in cardiac transplant recipients on cyclosporine with reduced corticosteroid use. Cleve Clin J Med 56:690, 1989

25. Dupont E: Molecular and cellular mechanisms of action of drugs used to modulate the immune response. Seminars in Thoracic and Cardiovascular Surgery 2:175, 1990

26. Hutter JA, Wallwork J, English TA: Management of rejection in heart transplant recipients: Does moderate rejection always require treatment? J Heart Transplant 9:87, 1990

27. Laufer G, Laczkovics A, Wollenek G et al: The progression of mild acute cardiac rejection evaluated by risk factor analysis. Transplantation 51:184, 1991

28. Radovancevic B, Birovljev S, Frazier OH: Treating cardiac allograft rejection: Present approach, analysis of 100 consecutive patients. J Heart Transplant 9:288, 1990

29. Miller LW: Treatment of cardiac allograft rejection with intravenous corticosteroids. J Heart Transplant 9:283, 1990

30. Hosenpud JD, Norman DJ, Pantely GA: Low-dose oral prednisone in the treatment of acute cardiac allograft rejection not associated with hemodynamic compromise. J Heart Transplant 9:292, 1990

31. Wahlers T, Heublein B, Cremer J et al: Treatment of rejection after heart transplantation: What dosage of pulsed steroids is necessary? J Heart Transplant 9:568, 1990

32. Deeb GM, Bolling SF, Steimle CN, Dawe JE, McKay AL, Richardson AM: A randomized prospective comparison of MALG with OKT3 for rescue therapy of acute myocardial rejection. Transplantation 51:180, 1991

33. Jones BM, Taylor FJ, Wright OM et al: Quality of life after heart transplantation in patients assigned to double- or triple-drug therapy. J Heart Transplant 9:392, 1990

34. Moore CK, Renlund DG, Rasmussen LG, O'Connnell JB: Long-term morbidity of cyclosporine with corticosteroid-free maintenance immunosuppression in cardiac transplantation. Transplant Proc 22:25, 1990

35. Winters GL, Kendall TJ, Radio SJ et al: Post-transplant obesity and hyperlipidemia: Major predictors of severity of coronary arteriopathy in failed human heart allografts. J Heart Transplant 9:364, 1990

36. Lewis RM, Van Buren CT, Radovancevic B et al: Impact of long-term cyclosporine immunosuppressive therapy on native kidneys versus renal allografts: Serial renal function in heart and kidney transplant recipients. Journal of Heart Lung Transplantation 10:63, 1991

37. Trull A, Hue K, Tan K et al: Cross-correlation of cyclosporine concentrations and biochemical measures of kidney and liver function in heart and heart-lung transplant recipients. Clin Chem 36:1474, 1990

38. Macris MP, Ford Eg, Van Buren CT, Frazier OH: Predictors of severe renal dysfunction after heart transplantation and intravenous cyclosporine therapy. J Heart Transplant 8:444, 1989

39. Bantle JP, Paller MS, Boudreau RJ, Olivari MT, Ferris TF: Long-term effects of cyclosporine on renal function in organ transplant recipients. J Lab Clin Med 115:233, 1990

40. Scherrer U, Vissing SF, Morgan BJ et al: Cyclosporine-induced sympathetic activation and hypertension after heart transplantation. N Engl J Med 323:693, 1990
41. Shapiro PA, Rutan GH, Thompson ME, Nigalye RL: Hypertension following orthotopic cardiac transplantation. Cardiovasc Clini 20:179, 1990
42. Farge D, Julien J, Amrein C et al: Effect of systemic hypertension on renal function and left ventricular hypertrophy in heart transplant recipients. J Am Coll Cardiol 15:1095, 1990
43. Spes CH, Angermann CE, Beyer RW et al: Increased incidence of cholelithiasis in heart transplant recipients receiving cyclosporine therapy. J Heart Transplant 9:404, 1990
44. Yee J, Petsikas D, Ricci MA, Guerraty A: General surgical procedures after heart transplantation. Can J Surg 33:185, 1990
45. DiSesa VJ, Kirkman RL, Tilney NL et al: Management of general surgical complications following cardiac transplantation. Arch Surg 124:539, 1989
46. Honda H, Barloon TJ, Franken EA Jr, Garneau RA, Smith JL: Clinical and radiologic features of malignant neoplasms in organ transplant recipients: cyclosporine-treated vs. untreated patients. American Journal of Roentgenology 154:271, 1990
47. Crandall BG, Gilbert EM, Renlund DG et al: A randomized trial of the immunosuppressive efficacy of vincristine in cardiac transplantation. Transplantation 50:34, 1990
48. Carrier M, Wild J, Pelletier LC, Copeland JG: Bromocriptine as an adjuvant to cyclosporine immunosuppression after heart transplantation. Ann Thorac Surg 49:129, 1990
49. Frist WH, Winterland AW, Gerhardt EB et al: Total lymphoid irradiation in heart transplantation: Adjunctive treatment for recurrent rejection. Ann Thorac Surg 48:863, 1989
50. Kaplan E, Dresdale AR, Diehl JT et al: Total lymphoid irradiation and discordant cardiac xenografts. J Heart Transplant 9:11, 1990
51. Todo S, Fung JJ, Starzl TE et al: Liver, kidney, and thoracic organ transplantation under FK 506. Ann Surg 212:295, 1990
52. Kapelanski DP, Perelman MJ, Faber LA, Paez DE, Rose EF, Behrendt DM: 15-Deoxysperguilan and primate heart transplantation. J Heart Transplant 9:668, 1990
53. Wood KJ, Morris PJ: Avenues for acquired immune tolerance. Seminars in Thoracic and Cardiovascular Surgery 2:189, 1990
54. Posselt AM, Barker CF, Tomaszewski JE, Markmann JF, Choti MA, Naji A: Induction of donor-specific unresponsiveness of intrathymic islet transplantation. Science 249:1293, 1990

Lauraine M. Stewart
Harry McCarthy
Judith A. Fabian

9 Use of Cardiopulmonary Bypass in Organ Transplantation

The basic principles of cardiopulmonary bypass are equally applicable for heart and heart–lung transplantation as for other cardiac procedures. Some modifications in technique are necessitated by the surgery and the physiology involved. Cardiopulmonary bypass may also be used during harvesting of the heart and lungs.

BASICS OF CARDIOPULMONARY BYPASS

The essential elements of the cardiopulmonary bypass circuit are the same despite differences in design and construction. Desaturated blood is drained from the venous system by gravity into a reservoir, from which it is passed through an oxygenator and heat exchanger and then pumped into the arterial circuit (Fig. 9-1).

The Oxygenator

The equipment currently in use reflects significant modifications and advances from the first clinically successful application of a mechanical heart and lung apparatus to cardiac surgery in 1954 by Gibbon.[1] The pre-

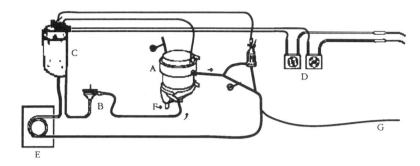

FIGURE 9-1. The essentials of the cardiopulmonary bypass apparatus. *A*, oxygenator; *B*, constrained vortex pump; *C*, cardiotomy and venous reservoir; *D*, cardiotomy suction; *E*, atrioventricular loop (in sterile sash); *F*, connection for thermal regulation; *G*, blood supply to cardioplegia system.

ferred method of oxygenating the blood has fluctuated between bubble oxygenators and membrane oxygenators.

Bubble oxygenators are made up of three different compartments: an oxygenating column, a defoaming compartment, and an arterial reservoir. Gas exchange occurs primarily in the oxygenating column, with a small amount of exchange occurring in the defoaming compartment. As the venous blood drains by gravity through the oxygenating column, a direct blood-gas interface occurs as oxygen is bubbled through the blood. The oxygen is passed through small holes in a plate or tube, and bubble size is determined by the size of the screen through which oxygen flows. The size of the bubble has a fundamental effect on the function of the device, as small bubbles give a larger surface area per unit of oxygen, thereby improving oxygenation. However, carbon dioxide removal depends on the volume of gas that ventilates the device. Low oxygen flows produce smaller bubbles and increase oxygenating capacity, whereas high flows result in more efficient carbon dioxide removal. A balance must be reached between well- controlled oxygenation and carbon dioxide elimination.

In the defoaming compartment, the arterialized blood is exposed to a large surface area of defoaming agent, which is a charged silicone polymer bonded to a polypropylene mesh. The charges are transferred to the foam, resulting in increased surface tension and reconstitution of the blood to its liquid form. A small amount of gas exchange occurs while the blood is passing through the defoamer. The defoaming capacity of the device must be great enough to handle the rated blood flow of the device so that the foam does not spill into the arterial line port. All units have a maximum flow rate that is determined by the manufacturer.

The arterial reservoir is the area in which the defoamed blood is collected before being pumped to the patient. The reservoir is designed so that residual microbubbles can float to the top, away from the outlet port located at the bottom of the reservoir. Flow of blood through the reservoir must be smooth so that any turbulence, which could generate further bubbles, is avoided. The maintenance of an adequate arterial reservoir level is important for a number of reasons: (1) the amount should be ample to allow the perfusionist a reasonable reaction time to stop the arterial pump should venous return be interrupted; (2) a greater volume in the reservoir increases the transit time of the blood, permits the absorption of smaller microbubbles, and allows larger macrobubbles to float up and away from the arterial port; and (3) the possibility of vortex formation and the entrainment of gas is minimized.

Membrane oxygenators seem to be safer and more physiologic than bubble oxygenators. Direct exposure of blood to gas is perceived to be damaging to blood, and it is believed that avoiding the risk of air embolism by not creating bubbles in the first place is preferable. In membrane oxygenators, blood and gas phases are completely separated, and gas exchange occurs through a synthetic membrane. The requisite large surface area is achieved by coiling or pleating the material or rolling it into a capillary configuration and packing the hollow fibers in a parallel fashion. In the most successful designs, gas flows through the capillaries surrounded by the blood. Although some blood-to-gas contact may occur at the initiation of cardiopulmonary bypass, a thin protein layer is quickly deposited over the pores to form a molecular membrane, which effectively separates the blood from the gas.

A true nonporous membrane oxygenator has been developed using a coiled silicone membrane. Gas transfer depends on the permeability of the membrane, the diffusion distance, and the driving pressure of the gas on either side of the membrane. Although no significant difference in blood trauma or in organ function is found with perfusions that last for 2 hours or less, membrane oxygenators have been shown to be superior to bubble oxygenators when prolonged perfusion is required.[2,3] Notable advantages include low blood trauma, low embolic risk, and the ability to vary gas exchange without changing blood flow rate. No studies compare bubble and membrane oxygenators for heart, heart–lung, or lung transplantation.

The Pump

Two types of pumps are currently in use during cardiopulmonary bypass: roller pumps and centrifugal pumps. Roller pumps, the most commonly used, consist of distensible rubber tubing with double-armed rollers that, when rotated, occlude the tubing against a backing plate, forcing the blood to flow in the direction of the rotation. The pump motor is designed to maintain a constant speed despite changes in pressure or resistance. Occlusiveness is adjusted to minimize blood trauma.

The constrained vortex-type pump operates through a series of concentric rotating cones, which produces a circular flow of blood within the pump and thereby generates a centrifugal force. The innermost cone spins by a magnetic connection to a drive shaft. Blood enters at the axis of the pump and exits at the periphery of the pump. If the pressure distal to the pump increases, then flow decreases. Output increases with pump speed. A flow meter placed between the patient and the pump must be used to determine actual flow rates.

The type of pump used depends primarily on the preference of the operator. The advantage of the roller head pump is that the pump flow is predictable depending on the pump speed. Disadvantages are that lines can be ruptured secondary to over-pressurization and that it is possible to pump large quantities of air. The centrifugal pump becomes effectively deprimed by gross air, although microbubbles can still be transmitted to the arterial line. The fact that pump speed does not necessarily reflect its output can be considered a negative feature.

Blood cell trauma that occurs during cardiopulmonary bypass is related to the physical stresses to which the blood is subjected in the system. Technical advances in both oxygenators and pumps have reduced these forces so that blood cell trauma is minimized. The most destructive aspect of the extracorporeal circuit is the suction apparatus for retrieving the blood that drains into the pericardial cavity. When air is aspirated with blood, a high level of trauma is thought to be the product of turbulent sheer stresses in the suction port.[4] The blood-gas and blood-tissue interfaces that result with suctioning from the operative field cause platelet activation and destruction.[5] Because the cardiotomy suction is a potent source of particulate emboli, micropore filters must be placed in the system to remove the emboli. These filters also contribute in part to platelet loss.

Cannulation

The techniques used for arterial and venous cannulation vary. Theoretically, any large artery or vein can be used for access. The arterial cannula is usually inserted into the ascending aorta. For cardiac transplantation, the recipient's ascending aorta may be cannulated in a slightly higher position than usual to facilitate access to the pericardial cavity. In transplant patients who have had previous cardiac surgery, the surgeon may elect to cannulate the femoral artery before sternotomy if the risk of hemorrhage from a difficult dissection is present or if the heart or aorta may have adhered to the underside of the sternum. This strategy provides a site for rapid infusion of blood or crystalloid in the event of major blood loss. If a catastrophe occurs while the chest is being opened, cannulation of the femoral artery and vein with initiation of partial bypass may be used as a temporizing measure while excessive bleeding is controlled. When cardiopulmonary bypass is required for single-lung transplantation, femorofemoral bypass is used for left lung transplantation and aortocaval bypass is used for right lung transplantation. Aortic dissection is more likely to occur with femoral cannulation.

When the surgical procedure does not require opening the right atrium, such as with coronary artery bypass grafting, a single, two-stage cannula that is designed to sit in the midcavity of the right atrium with the distal portion in the inferior vena cava is frequently used. Venous drainage, including coronary sinus return, is achieved via the inferior vena cava and the right atrium.[6] For cardiac transplantation, where most of the atrium is excised, the inferior and superior vena cavae are cannulated separately (bicaval cannulation), and ligatures are placed around the cavae to prevent drainage of venous blood into the atrium. Furthermore, no air can enter the venous side of the bypass circuit to create an air lock.

To achieve satisfactory drainage from a femoral vein, it is necessary to pass the cannula beyond the external iliac vein into the high inferior vena cava. Even if this positioning cannot be achieved, it is still possible to go on partial bypass, open the chest, and establish right atrial drainage in an emergency situation.

Thermal Regulation

Cooling and rewarming are controlled by heat exchangers during cardiopulmonary bypass. Cardiac hypothermia is achieved by systemic cooling with cold cardiopulmonary bypass perfusate, instilling cold cardioplegic solution into the coronary arteries in an antegrade or retrograde fashion, and topically cooling with an iced solution.[7,8] Although inadequate alone, systemic hypothermia contributes to myocardial preservation by preventing rewarming of the heart.

Cardioplegia

Cold cardioplegic solutions used to arrest the heart are either crystalloid- or blood-based. Constituents of the solutions vary from one institution to another. Generally, cardioplegic solutions use potassium chloride (15–30 mEq/L) to achieve immediate cardiac arrest. Mannitol or albumin are used to adjust osmolality and decrease cellular edema; buffering agents are added to counteract acidosis; and magnesium is used to block ischemic Ca^{++} entry into the cell. A number of other additives have been tried, such as procaine, lidocaine, or nitroglycerin, to abolish vasoconstriction, and calcium channel blockers have been tried to abolish vasoconstriction and prevent ischemic Ca^{++} entry. Addition of the free radical scavengers catalase and superoxide dismutase has been demonstrated to provide better cardiac performance after reperfusion in canine transplanted hearts.[9]

In the presence of severe coronary artery disease, maximal uniform delivery of the cold cardioplegic solution may be difficult to accomplish.[10] Because only hearts with normal coronary arteries are accepted for transplantation, delivery of the cardioplegia may be more reliably homogeneous.

EFFECTS OF CARDIOPULMONARY BYPASS

The artificial environment of cardiopulmonary bypass causes multiple major violations of the normal physiologic state. In a recent comprehensive review, Knudsen and Anderson surveyed evidence relative to immunologic derangements that occur during cardiopulmonary bypass. They divided cellular and humoral changes into two subsets: normal host defenses against infection, and systemic inflammatory responses. They noted that immediate or shortly delayed immunodepression was evidenced by decreases in serum immunoglobulin concentrations and impairment of serum opsonizing capacity. Host defense reactions to infection were all depressed either during or immediately after bypass. Generalized inflammatory reactions, which consisted of complement activation with generation of anaphylatoxins C3a and C5a, stimulation of polymorphonuclear leukocytes, and release of reactive oxygen species and lysosomal enzymes, also occurred. These immunologic changes appear to play a significant role in postoperative morbidity.[11] Further data are needed to thoroughly understand the clinical significance of these observed changes; however, the impact on a transplant recipient is most certainly compounded by immunosuppressive therapy to prevent rejection of the donor organ.

Hematologic disorders are also possible consequences of cardiopulmonary bypass. In a review of the etiologies of mediastinal bleeding after cardiac surgery, Czer summarized the hemostatic derangements that occur from exposure of the patient's blood to extracorporeal circulation.[12] Platelet dysfunction was regarded as the most important disorder that resulted in significant blood loss. Platelet activation and damage, as reflected in elevated beta-thromboglobulin levels, have been reported regardless of the type of circuit or oxygenator used. Complement activation, as well as the direct activation of platelets by bypass components, has been implicated as being instrumental in platelet dysfunction. The degree of platelet dysfunction has been found to be proportional to the length of cardiopulmonary bypass, the depth of hypothermia, and the extent of reinfusion of blood after uncontrolled cardiotomy suctioning. Patients for cardiac transplantation may have additional bleeding problems imposed by the presence of preoperative liver congestion.

Cardiopulmonary bypass is associated with a stress response in both children and adults that may contribute to its damaging effects. Reves has proposed that attenuation of the stress response by various anesthetic techniques could improve outcome and influence the postoperative course.[13] The patient's ability to compensate for the abnormal physiologic environment to which he or she has been exposed is a major factor in determination of outcome of cardiopulmonary bypass. Poor overall condition would appear to have a significant influence, and the ill transplant patient may be at risk for increased morbidity.

ORGAN PROCUREMENT AND PRESERVATION

Long-distance harvesting has increased the availability of donor organs.[14] However, the increased ischemic time involved has necessitated development of methods to protect those organs from ischemic damage. Organ preservation is achieved by reducing metabolic demand and increasing the supply of oxygen and nutrients.

Hypothermia

Preservation of the excised donor heart was initially achieved by simple hypothermia using cold saline.[15] Until recently, this method was still used by the group at the Medical College of Virginia. Although hypothermia decreases metabolic demand, activity does not cease entirely, and the organ is still at risk for ischemic injury.

Hypothermia and Cardioplegia

Most centers use a combination of topical hypothermia and cold, hyperkalemic cardioplegia to achieve donor heart protection. The high concentration of potassium inhibits metabolism by depolarizing the cell membrane. Other cardioplegic agents have also been under investigation.[16]

Total Body Perfusion

Cardiopulmonary bypass is not only used for reimplantation of the donor heart into the recipient, but cardiopulmonary bypass with profound hypothermia has also been used to harvest multiple organs from a single donor. Although other successful preservation techniques have been described, the advantages of this one include a gradual and complete cooling of the organs and less hemodynamic compromise when organs are dissected from an unstable donor. The technique of cardiopulmonary bypass with profound hypothermia is the preferred method for heart–lung procurement. Because it is equally as successful as standard techniques used in the procurement of other organs, its use for heart–lung procurement does not preclude harvesting other organs.

The availability of portable bypass units permits procurement of organs from donors located in distant hospitals. A perfusionist from the transplant center accompanies the surgical team to the donor hospital. The list of supplies and equipment required is not large (Table 9-1). With appropriate planning, the portable perfusion set-up may be packed into a fairly compact unit that can easily be accommodated by the small jets used for long-distance transport of donor organs (Fig. 9-2).

The technique consists of placing an arterial cannula into the femoral artery for inflow and a two-stage venous cannula into the right atrium or inferior vena cava for outflow, using standard surgical procedures to institute cardiopulmonary bypass.[17] After bypass has been ini-

TABLE 9-1. Equipment Needed for Heart–Lung Procurement Using Portable Cardiopulmonary Bypass

Equipment	Out	Return
Oxygenator and holder	X	X
Cardiotomy holder	X	X
Bypass tubing pack	X	
Venous bag and ⅜″ tubing adapters	X	
(2) 24″ pieces of ⅜″ x ³⁄₃₂″ tubing	X	
6-foot piece of ⅜″ x ³⁄₃₂″ tubing in case lines are dropped	X	
Extra small line with one-way valve	X	
Unsterile vacuum line	X	
(2) Centrifugal pump heads	X	X
Pump (check for fully charged battery)	X	X
Flow probe	X	X
Extension cord and 2 adaptor cords for centrifugal pump	X	X
Cooler	X	X
Water pump and lines in cooler	X	X
Temperature box (check batteries) and 2 probes	X	X
Oxygen regulator	X	X
(2) Screw clamps	X	X
(8) Tubing clamps	X	X
(3) Bottles of heparin (1000 U/mL) and syringe with needle	X	
Tie bands and banding gun	X	X
Scissors	X	X
Flexible intracardiac suction tip	X	
(2) Two-stage venous cannulae	X	
(2) 24F flexible arterial cannulae	X	
(2) Connectors, ⅜″ x ⅜″ with luer lock	X	
(2) Connectors, ⅔″ x ⅜″ with luer lock	X	

tiated, preliminary dissection of the mediastinal and abdominal organs can be accomplished during cooling. Additional cannulation of the portal vein, abdominal aorta, and the inferior vena cava may be performed to perfuse the liver, kidneys, and pancreas with the flush solutions preferred by the individual transplant teams that are retrieving those organs. The use of an asanguinous prime decreases viscosity and enhances flow to all the organs. Temperature is lowered to about 10° to 15°C, at which point bypass is discontinued, and the heart and lungs are removed en bloc. By this time, the abdominal organs have been flushed with crystalloid solutions and are prepared for dissection. Organs procured by this technique have functioned as well or better than those retrieved by more conventional methods.[18,19]

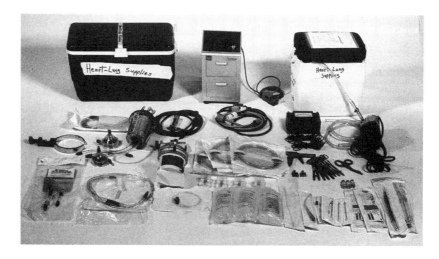

A

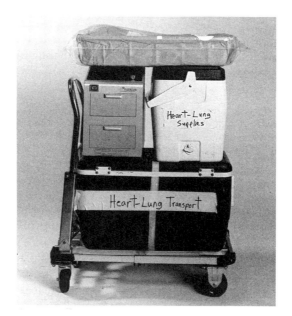

B

FIGURE 9-2. The equipment required for heart–lung procurement using portable cardiopulmonary bypass. *A*, The equipment has been spread out for inventory. *B*, The equipment is compact enough to be stowed on a small jet.

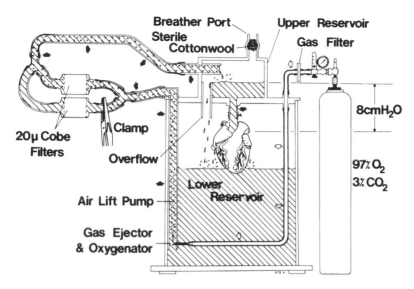

FIGURE 9-3.   Hypothermic perfusion apparatus for the excised heart. (Wicomb WN, Cooper DKC: Storage of the donor heart. In Cooper DKC, Novitsky D (eds): The Transplantation and Replacement of Thoracic Organs, p. 55. Boston, Kluwer Academic Publishers, 1990)

Extracorporeal Hypothermic Perfusion

Continuous hypothermic perfusion of excised heart (Fig. 9-3) and heart–lung preparations (Fig. 9-4) has been used in experimental animals in an attempt to extend the available ischemic period.[20-23] Theoretically, this perfusion is advantageous because, in addition to providing depression of metabolic function, it provides a continuous supply of oxygen and nutrients as well as removal of waste products. Although this system has not proved advantageous in clinical practice, refinements in composition of perfusate solutions may make its use more feasible.[24]

Hypothermic Flush Perfusion

Most solid organs are preserved for transplantation by means of a simple hypothermic flush solution followed by static hypothermic storage. Initially, EuroCollins solution modified by the addition of magnesium sulfate was used (Table 9-2);[25] however, other crystalloid and colloid solu-

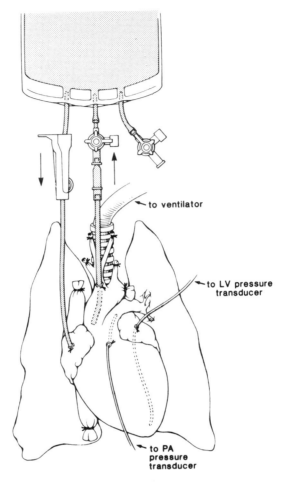

to ventilator

to LV pressure
transducer

to PA
pressure
transducer

FIGURE 9-4. The autoperfused heart–lung preparation. *PA,* pulmonary artery; *LV,* left ventricle. *(Kaplan E, Diehl JT, Peterson MB et al: Extended ex vivo preservation of the heart and lungs. J Thorac Cardiovasc Surg 100:687, 1990)*

tions have also been developed.[26–28] Cold autologous blood modified by the addition of albumin, mannitol, and buffers has also been used.[29,30] Flush solutions have been further modified by the addition of platelet-activating factor antagonist; free radical scavengers such as dimethylthiourea, liposomal superoxide dismutase, and catalase; calcium channel blockers; deferoxamine (an iron chelator that inhibits formation of oxygen-derived free radicals); and indomethacin.[24,31–35]

TABLE 9-2. Composition of Modified
EuroCollins Solution

Component	Amount
KH_2PO_4	2.05 g/L
K_2HPO_4	7.40 g/L
KCl	1.12 g/L
$NaHCO_3$	0.84 g/L
$MgSO_4$	1.00 g/L
Glucose	38.5 g/L
pH	7.3–7.4

CONCLUSION

Cardiopulmonary bypass is an integral part of heart, heart–lung, and single-lung transplantation. Its extension to organ procurement has enabled the excision of multiple organs in a bloodless field with improved organ function. Function of solid organs has also improved with the use of various hypothermic flush solutions.

References

1. Gibbon JH Jr: Application of a mechanical heart and lung apparatus to cardiac surgery. Minn Med 37:171, 1954
2. Clark RE, Beauchamp RA, Magrath RA et al: Comparison of bubble and membrane oxygenators in short and long perfusions. J Thorac Cardiovasc Surg 78:655, 1979
3. Van Oeveren W, Kazatchkine MD, Descamps-Latscha B et al: Deleterious effects of cardiopulmonary bypass: A prospective study of bubble versus membrane oxygenation. J Thorac Cardiovasc Surg 89:888, 1985
4. Okies JE, Goodnight SH, Litchford B et al: Effects of infusion of cardiotomy suction blood during extracorporeal circulation for coronary artery bypass surgery. J Thorac Cardiovasc Surg 74:440, 1977
5. Boonstra PW, Van Imhoff GW, Eysman L et al: Reduced platelet activation and improved hemostasis after controlled cardiotomy suction. J Thorac Cardiovasc Surg 89:900, 1985
6. Riley JB, Hardin SB, Winn BA et al: In vitro comparison of cavoatrial (dual stage) cannulae for use during cardiopulmonary bypass. Perfusion 1:197, 1986
7. Landymore RW, Tice D, Trehan N et al: Importance of topical hypothermia to ensure uniform myocardial cooling during coronary artery bypass. J Thorac Cardiovasc Surg 82:832, 1981
8. Grover F, Fewel JG, Ghidoni JJ et al: Does lower systemic pressure enhance cardioplegic myocardial protection? J Thorac Cardiovasc Surg 81:11, 1981

9. Bando K, Senoo Y: Oxygen-derived free radical damage in canine heart transplantation. J Surg Res 46:152, 1989
10. Hilton CJ, Teubl W, Acker M et al: Inadequate cardioplegic protection with obstructed coronary arteries. Ann Thorac Surg 28:323, 1979
11. Knudson F, Anderson LW: Immunological aspects of cardiopulmonary bypass. J Cardiothor Anesth 4:245, 1990
12. Czer LSC: Mediastinal bleeding after cardiac surgery: etiologies, diagnostic considerations, and blood conservation methods. Journal of Cardiothoracic Anesthesia 3:760, 1989
13. Reves JG: Anesthesia and cardiopulmonary bypass. Anesth Analg (suppl) 93:10, 1991
14. Thomas FT, Szentpetery SS, Mammana RE, Wolfgang TC, Lower RR: Long-distance transportation of human hearts for transplantation. Ann Thorac Surg 26:344, 1978
15. Lower RR, Stofer RC, Hurley EJ, Dong E Jr, Cohn RB, Shumway NE: Successful homotransplantation of the canine heart after anoxic preservation for seven hours. Am J Surg 104:302, 1962
16. Mollhoff T, Sukehiro S, Van Aken H, Flameng W: Long-term preservation of baboon hearts: Effects of hypothermic ischemic and cardioplegic arrest on high-energy phosphate content. Circulation (suppl) 82:264, 1990
17. Baumgartner WA, Williams GM, Fraser CD Jr et al: Cardiopulmonary bypass with profound hypothermia. Transplantation 47:123, 1989
18. Hardesty RL, Griffith BP: Procurement for combined heart–lung transplantation: Bilateral thoracotomy with sternal transection, cardiopulmonary bypass, and profound hypothermia. J Thorac Cardiovasc Surg 89:795, 1985
19. Baumgartner WA, Traill TA, Cameron DE, Fonger JD, Birenbaum IB, Reitz BA: Unique aspects of heart and lung transplantation exhibited in the 'domino-donor' operation. JAMA 261:3121, 1989
20. Wicomb WN, Cooper DKC: Storage of the donor heart. In Cooper DKC, Novitsky D (eds): The Transplantation and Replacement of Thoracic Organs, p. 55. Boston, Kluwer Academic Publishers, 1990
21. Kioka Y, Tago M, Bando K et al: Twenty-four hours isolated heart preservation by perfusion method with oxygenated solution containing perfluorochemicals and albumin. J Heart Transplant 5:437, 1986
22. Cooper DKC, Wicomb WN, Barnard CN: Storage of the donor heart by a portable hypothermic perfusion system: Experimental development and clinical experience. J Heart Transplant 2:104, 1983
23. Kresh JY, Brockman SK: Autoperfusing ectothermic heart–lung preservation system. Journal of Investigational Surgery 2:281, 1989
24. Kaplan E, Diehl JT, Peterson MB et al: Extended ex vivo preservation of the heart and lungs. J Thorac Cardiovasc Surg 100:687, 1990
25. Jamieson SW, Stinson EB, Oyer PE, Baldwin JC, Shumway NE: Operative technique for heart–lung transplantation. J Thorac Cardiovasc Surg 87:930, 1984
26. Wang G, Reader J, Hynd J, Pepper J: Improved heart and lung preservation in a rat model. Transpl Int 19903:206, 1990
27. Naka Y, Shirakura R, Matsuda H et al: Canine heart–lung transplantation after 24-hour hypothermic preservation. Eur J Cardiothorac Surg 4:499, 1990

28. McGoldrick JP, Scott JP, Smyth R, Higenbottam T, Wallwork J: Early graft function after heart–lung transplantation. J Heart Transplant 9:693, 1990
29. Hakim M, Higenbottam T, Bethune D et al: Selection and procurement of combined heart and lung grafts for transplantation. J Thorac Cardiovasc Surg 95:474, 1988
30. Locke TJ, Hooper TL, FLecknell PA, McGregor CG: Preservation of the lung: Comparison of flush perfusion with cold modified blood and core cooling by cardiopulmonary bypass. J Heart Lung Transplant 10:1, 1991
31. Conte JV Jr, Katz NM, Wallace RB, Foegh ML: Long-term lung preservation with the PAF antagonist BN 52021. Transplantation 51:1152, 1991
32. Lambert CJ Jr, Egan TM, Detterbeck FC, Keagy BA, Wilcox BR: Enhanced pulmonary function using dimethylthiourea for twelve-hour lung preservation. Ann Thorac Surg 51:924, 1991
33. Detterbeck FC, Keagy BA, Paull DE, Wilcox BR: Oxygen free radical scavengers decrease reperfusion injury in lung transplantation. Ann Thorac Surg 50:204, 1990
34. Cremer J, Jurmann M, Dammenhayn L et al: Oxygen free radical scavengers to prevent pulmonary reperfusion injury after heart–lung transplantation. J Heart Transplant 8:330, 1989
35. Pickford MA, Green CJ, Sarathchandra P, Fryer PR: Ultrastructural changes in rat lungs after 48 h cold storage with and without reperfusion. International Journal of Experimental Pathology 71:513, 1990

Roger Balk

Ethical Issues in Organ Transplantation as Standard Therapy

10

"... we believe that the largest and perhaps most enduring significance of organ transplantation and dialysis lies in the ethical and existential questions they raise. Problems of uncertainty, meaning, life and
death, scarcity, justice, equity, solidarity, and intervention in the
human condition are all evoked by these therapeutic interventions.
Transplantation and dialysis have played an important role in making
such moral and metaphysical concerns more visible and legitimate in
present day medicine."[1]

Some of our most cherished symbols of finitude have been
destroyed or radically modified as the result of technological innova-
tions. Our image of the heart, breathing, what constitutes death, or even
an essential body part has had to change, and with it have changed the
personal and social sensibilities and structures that these images have
provided to understand the moral and existential implications of our finitude. This challenge does not extend only to those vestiges of traditional
religious life that remain in the last decade of the 20th century. For example, it is difficult to find words to describe accurately the condition and
status of a dead potential organ donor. Increasing evidence shows that
individuals who receive transplants have some difficulty with their
resulting body image.[2] It is still the frequent feeling in intensive care units
that stopping life support in a brain-dead patient is causing his or her
death. So the comments of Fox and Swazey as they summarized the early

years of organ transplantation still hold, even though this technology has progressed to the point of being a standard treatment.

TRANSPLANT DONORS

Where Do We Get Organs for Transplantation?

The first successful donors were identical twins of the recipient. The limited number of circumstances under which such exchange could be undertaken made its value largely an indication that under the right circumstances transplantation was possible.[3] The extension of this procedure to include kidneys from unrelated cadaver donors depended on the development of therapies to prevent rejection of foreign tissue by the recipient.

The invention of the respirator made it possible to preserve an organ in vivo until such time as it was required. The use of this device created other more complicated problems. How was one to determine that a potential donor was legally dead?[4] How was one to overcome all of the culturally determined practices and feelings associated with death determination and respect for the newly deceased in order to make organ harvesting an accepted practice?[5] How might the law be reinterpreted, since it normally recognized cessation of heartbeat and breathing as the indication of death?[6] The Harvard Criteria for brain death determination made cadaveric organ recovery possible on the scale necessary to support the development of multiorgan transplantation.[7] Although the answer may not be clear-cut, the impetus for the development of the Harvard Criteria seems to have come largely from the needs of the promising new transplantation technology to solve the cadaveric donor problem. We should note, however, that creation of the respirator in itself provoked the need for another way to determine death, otherwise the practice of "pulling the plug" could have been regarded as a deliberate act of killing a patient connected to this mechanical life support. Most states have amended their criminal codes to permit alternative means of determining death and thereby prevent the chaos that followed attempts to find doctors guilty of murder because they used brain-death criteria to allow for the removal of vital organs.[8]

Death determination by the Harvard Criteria itself placed considerable emphasis on the trustworthiness of technology. The use of the electroencephalogram (EEG) in certifying the absence of all brain activity was accepted from the beginning. In the case of children, this test has been supplemented with cerebral blood flow analysis. Acceptance of these standards meant recognition that technology could provide a fail-safe means of certifying legal death in a heart-beating corpse and allow for the harvest of organs from cadavers.

Creating a Dependable Supply of Organs

The existence of the knowledge and technology necessary for the creation of the cadaver donor led almost immediately to another problem: how to create a system to assure their supply. Initially, individual transplant centers began to develop referral networks, sensitizing colleagues at nearby hospitals to the need for cadaver donors and helping them to develop the skills necessary to identify and maintain potential donors. By 1968, "renal banks" had been organized in Boston and Los Angeles. Although the supply of organs, mostly kidneys, was not large, it served the needs of the slowly increasing numbers of transplant centers. By the mid-1970s, limits to the supply caused the Center for Disease Control to study the numbers of donors that could be available if an efficient system for their identification and allocation existed.[9,10] The fact that rejection remained an unsolved problem for transplantation of other organs, particularly the heart, kept the demand at a level that could still be handled by the systems developed in individual transplant institutions. With the advent of cyclosporine in 1980, the rejection problem became manageable for a wide variety of transplanted organs, and the need for a better system for donor organ allocation arose. The first organizations were geographically limited to insure distribution within the limits of ischemic time for each organ. Exchange among contiguous regions was facilitated through distribution of waiting lists, telephone communication, and, finally, integrated computer systems.

The complex system that has been created to facilitate the identification and retrieval of human organs has been based on the notion of an elaborate gift exchange. This notion has been altered with changes in technology that made the cadaveric donor the major source of organ supply and has emerged under the more impersonal category of altruism. The sophisticated system of organized charity in the United States was adapted to the needs of organizing a voluntary organ procurement system. However, this principle, which supports the system for obtaining body parts by limiting organs available to those that are given, also produces a number of challenges to its efficiency. Basically, to work well, every potential donor must be identified and "asked" to give his or her organs.

Ambivalence on the part of hospital staff who must work with these people and their families is reflected in the results of studies, which indicate that a major contributor to the donor shortage is the failure of hospitals to identify potential donors at the point at which they can possibly become actual donors.[11]

In a recent study in Quebec, 224 neurologists and neurosurgeons, 202 administrators and medical directors of intensive care units, as well as 1997 staff nurses from emergency rooms and intensive care units were polled as to their attitudes toward a number of issues related to the identification and care of potential organ donors. While an overwhelming majority (85%) was favorable to the concept of organ donation, they were almost equally of the feeling that asking for the organs and coping with their care were burdens that they preferred not to have.

Legislation to require routine inquiry about organ donation has been attempted as a solution to this reluctance to approach families.[12] Required Request or Required Consideration legislation makes the system no longer dependent on personal initiative by relegating it to one of those bureaucratic procedures brought about by death. It is not clear that this problem is amenable to an administrative fix, since recent studies have indicated that large numbers of potential donors go unreported to those organ procurement organizations in jurisdictions that have required request laws.

Many advocates of modifying the organ procurement system have recommended that the voluntary approach be modified or abolished altogether. Several European jurisdictions have enacted Presumed Consent laws, which assume that everyone has given consent to his or her organs being used unless he or she has specifically recorded otherwise. The principle that underlies this legislation is that, once a person has died, his or her body parts may be claimed by the state, since they are not owned by the relatives. In practice, doctors in all countries that use this system still require approval by the family for organ donation.[13,14] What these examples illustrate is that activating the potential of brain-dead persons to become organ donors requires much more than the technological capacity to do so.

Meeting the Demand for More Organs

A more fundamental issue has often gone unnoticed. The extent to which the establishment of transplantation as standard treatment requires meeting the demand for organs at individual transplant centers at whatever level they have established as current need has the effect of disguising wide variations in selection criteria, particularly with regard to what constitutes valid criteria for retransplantation. All that is seen on the computer is a name on a waiting list at the appropriate level of priority. A discussion about allocation separate from the question of organ supply is needed.

It is not surprising that the success of transplantation has made the search for additional sources of vital organs a major concern. Three of these efforts require some consideration.

Paying for Organs

The potential for increasing use of living nonrelated donors has led, in some parts of the world, to the introduction of paying people to become donors. This practice has been most commonly used for kidney transplants. Because this method is against the law in the United States, we have been quick to raise concerns about exploitation, particularly when such individuals are from the third world or of limited income.[15,16]

The Extension of Organ Donation by Living Donors to Other Body Organs such as Lung and Liver

Although clearly experimental, this practice has proved in limited use to be clinically feasible. It obviously involves considerably greater risk to the donor and raises the question of what limits should be placed on persons eligible to provide a portion of their own organs. At the present time, it has been limited to parent–child relationships and, presumably by extension, child to parent. Other family configurations appear to be possible as well, since they have been legitimized by considerable experience. Once we leave the family circle and its traditional practices of mutual support, the issue becomes clouded, particularly because of the much higher risks to the donor.

The Use of Xenografts

The most significant disruption of current transplantation practice is provided by the prospect of xenografts and the potential for overriding the problems of histocompatibility through transgenic manipulation of the animal donor. The donor shortage would be alleviated because nonhumans would be effectively indistinguishable from humans from the point of view of histocompatibility. Problems that become immediately obvious are: (1) allocation, who gets the human organ and who gets the xenograft when we are not sure if one is preferable from the view of outcome; (2) animal rights, can we justify the raising and killing of thousands of animals for the purposes of transplantation; and (3) cost, can we afford the expenditures on this health care procedure that would result when the limits on outlay provided by the natural shortage of donor organs would no longer exist.

Organ Donation as a Matter of Public Policy

Critical decisions relative to public policy about transplantation have been dominated by a small group of medical specialists. In spite of the fact that organ donation and allocation have been the subject of extensive hearings in Congress, studied extensively by a number of public and private research projects, and administered by the United Network for Organ Sharing (UNOS), the rules of which are government regulations, it has been extremely difficult to develop representation on governing boards of both regional organ procurement organizations and UNOS itself in which transplant doctors do not hold the effective power. While this fact is not surprising, given that success of organ transplantation is the result of the efforts of research scientists and medical practitioners, it is not obvious that this practice should continue. At some point in its development, transplantation must become subject to scrutiny from the viewpoint of social ethics and public policy.

In view of where we are today, a number of questions need to be asked about who is making macro level decisions that determine the way the transplant industry is run. Why should transplant surgeons and physicians continue to dominate the boards of directors of most local organ procurement organizations or have such a large block of the representation at the decision-making levels of UNOS, when most of the issues related to organ donation or allocation are not technical, but social and political? The philosophy of medicine that supports the decision to turn the dying process into an opportunity for organ donation affects other members of the medical profession far more than it does transplant surgeons and physicians; yet, it is rare for critical care physicians, neurologists, or neurosurgeons to have much input into the development of policies that relate to organ donation.[17] The unwillingness to control the expansion of transplant centers in a rational way suggests that values other than those of the best use of resources or the care of patients determine the increase in the numbers of transplant centers.[18]

Allocating the Number of Organs Available

It is a standard refrain that the shortage of organ donors continues to restrict the treatment potential of transplantation.[19] It is also an excuse to escape the ethical dilemma of whether we are allocating organs in a fair and just manner because the present system is often justified as driven by the organ shortage.

How important is it that an organ be given to the person who is likely to live the longest? In the case of kidney transplants, for which the significance of the HLA system was discovered, it has been assumed that the best match between donor and recipient tissue would always enhance graft life. Although this assumption may have been the case before the cyclosporine era, current data are unclear whether much is gained by running the allocation system on the basis of HLA match. At any given time, the decision of the Board of Directors of UNOS on this subject is a function of which advocates of which point of view happen to be in the majority. Scientific evidence does not make a definitive contribution toward resolving whether this elaborate and costly matching system is a fair and just way to distribute kidneys.[20]

The issue has more to it than just this debate. Selecting potential recipients for crossmatch based on HLA matching favors those with the frequently occurring HLA-Ag. Such matching policies are especially punitive to blacks, who have different HLA-Ag frequencies, since it deprives them of equal access to most of the 75% of kidneys that come from other racial or ethnic groups.[21] To justify the present method of allocation, which is heavily weighted in favor of the white, European portion of the population, would require arguing that the length of graft survival be the sole criteria for allocating kidneys.

Another method of determining priority in organ allocation has been the practice of giving precedence to the most urgent patient on the list. While this method responds to the concern to help those who will not survive without an intervention, it is not necessarily a way to make the best use of high technology. Although advocates of this practice must assume that risk of mortality is highly predictable, the absence of clear clinical standards for specifying the comparative status of all patients with highest priority means that undocumented criteria are clouding the application of specific standards of justice and fairness. For example, institutions that employ mechanical cardiac support devices have been able to claim absolute priority for their patients when a heart becomes available. What emerges is evidence that medical criteria have become defined and applied to the allocation of organs in a nonscientific way and that the system would be better off if a demystification of the criteria took place.

The absence of universal access to transplantation on the basis of established medical criteria precludes the existence of a fair system of organ allocation because no such restriction on accepting organs from those too poor to qualify for a transplant exists. This fact is particularly offensive when we see others who are able to procure one or more retransplants because they can afford to be placed on a public waiting list from the confines of a private hospital. The recent steps taken by the State of Oregon which proposed removing transplantation from those procedures available to people on Medicaid illustrates the ironies that emerge in the present system.

A fair system of allocation must possess at least these qualities: (1) it must provide criteria that make selection standards equal so that positions on the waiting list portray similar health and risk states; (2) the waiting list must include, as nearly as possible, all patients likely to benefit from a transplant, making it representative of those for whom a fair and just outcome is desired; (3) ability to pay cannot be included as a condition of selection because all those who receive this procedure are beneficiaries of a public subsidy without which almost no one could afford the procedure; and (4) everyone on the list should have an equal chance of receiving the next organ.

TRANSPLANT RECIPIENTS

Screening and Selection of Potential Recipients

The rationale for current screening and selection of potential recipients is to identify patients who will have less likelihood of surviving another year without transplantation than dying of the transplant procedure. In addition, screening identifies those who have other systemic problems likely to jeopardize their survival after they receive an organ. An important aim of the screening process is to prevent deaths in the perioperative period caused by patients who are too sick to survive major surgery.[22]

The length of the waiting list may be affecting selection decisions. The temptation to manipulate the psychosocial criteria that are used to determine a person's fitness to cope with the continued physical challenges to his well-being may be great. Among the more controversial of these standards are those that attempt to decide how previous lifestyles, such as use of alcohol and tobacco, should affect eligibility for transplantation. The right of a selection committee to require reasonable indication on the part of a potential recipient that he or she has the responsibility to control or end an aberrant lifestyle has been upheld, but it is clear that this right is greatly restricted.[23] The underlying issue is whether allocation concerns due to organ shortage are altering standards used to determine a person's fitness to undergo organ transplantation in a way that avoids issues of fairness and justice in the allocation of available organs.

Quality of Life

The quality of life of kidney and heart transplant recipients has been subjected to extensive review.[24,25] Results of surveys suggest that the level of health enjoyed by most kidney and heart transplant patients was sufficiently high to satisfy comparison with other medical procedures and even so-called normal people.[26] What has become obvious to those who have been able to observe heart transplant recipients over an extended time period is that these studies have not been able to uncover what life is really like after transplantation.

The dilemma of the transplant patients is how to adjust to a situation in which they are neither dying nor cured. Transplantation trades an acute end-stage disease state for a chronic-illness state. Every recipient is dependent on long-term care by a specialized health care team. In the preoperative teaching, it is emphasized to prospective recipients that they will not be able to cope with the dangers of rejection, infection, and so forth, unless they are willing to use their expertise at any time, day or night, to determine that something is not right. Many recipients eventually acquire a sense of what their new body life is like and are able to sense when potential trouble is at hand. Others never manage to comprehend their new state and mechanically perform the required daily rituals (i.e., recording blood pressure, temperature, pulse, medications). Quality of life studies have generally ignored the adaptive mechanisms the patient develops to meet these challenges.

Differences between physician and patient assessments of health status make it difficult to know the reasonable expectations for rehabilitation of transplant recipients. An informal study of 100 patients who received heart transplants since 1985 at Royal Victoria Hospital in Montreal indicated that 90% were able to assume full activity. However, a high percentage of the same patients indicated that they had significantly impaired short-term memory, capacity for concentration, ability to deal with stress, and ability to control aggressiveness. Anxiety levels continued at much the same level as when they were put on the transplant waiting list. Although physical recovery did not seem to be affected by age, the psychological symptoms seemed to be exacerbated in the older person.

Generally speaking, private insurance programs have been a major deterrent to transplant recipients resuming their previous occupation. They retain coverage only so long as they continue their disabled status. The whole purpose of the transplant enterprise becomes subverted if major limitations are placed on the patient's return to normal working status by life and health insurance coverage limitations.

Creating a New Person

It is not inaccurate to think of the effects of organ transplantation as creating a new person. The demands of the technology initiate from the screening period onward an intense involvement of the transplant team in the personal lives of each patient and his or her family. It is almost impossible to draw a meaningful distinction between the medical and personal problems a patient experiences. The time spent waiting for a new organ is a period of excruciating anxiety for patients and their families. The anxiety of waiting for an organ is replaced by the worry that it will fail. Normal social life and the needs of other members of the family get put on hold, a fact that all too often becomes permanent.

Many adults report that their sense of self, or body image, has been permanently altered by the transplant.[27] Studies, including those that make use of projective tests, suggest this experience is very real. What we do not know is the mechanism by which this event becomes adaptive or maladaptive. Of more concern is the fact that we know little about whether this experience is also found among children who receive transplantation.

Relationships with spouses, significant others, and children are permanently affected by the experience of transplantation. Sexual dysfunction continues to be prevalent among those who receive new hearts. Other members of the family wonder when it will be their turn to receive some attention. Although many of these experiences have been reported in some detail by those who study the long-term effects of chronic illness on the family configuration, it is important to remember that we are creating a chronic illness state and calling it restoration to physical health.

CONCLUSION

The dramatic effects of organ transplantation have given it symbolic quality. It represents the achievements of the technological transformation that has affected medical care today. The fact that it is, in effect, a process of buying time forces us to consider the ways in which the use of technology instantly requires placing value on persons and acts. It reveals how just and fair we believe it is necessary for our society to be.

References

1. Fox RC, Swazey JP: In: The Courage to Fail, 2nd ed, p. 1. Chicago, University of Chicago Press, 1, 1969
2. Castelnuovo-Tadesco P: Psychological inhibitions of changes in body image. In Levy N (ed): Psychonephrology. I. Psychological factors in Hemodialysis and Transplantation, p. 219. New York, Plenum, 1981
3. Merrill JP, Murray JE, Harrison JH, Guild WR: Successful homotransplantation of the human kidney between identical twins. JAMA 160:277, 1956
4. Ramsey P: On updating death. In Cutler D (ed): Updating Life and Death, p. 16. Boston, Beacon Press, 1969
5. Youngner SJ: Psychosocial and ethical implications of organ retrieval. New Engl J Med 313:321, 1985
6. Capron AM, Kass LR: A statutory definition of the standards for determining human death: An appraisal and a proposal. University of Pennsylvania Law Review 121:87 1972
7. Ad Hoc Committee of the Harvard Medical School. A definition of irreversible coma. JAMA 205:85, 1968.
8. Tucker *v.* Lower. No. 2831 (Richmond, VA). Law & Equity Court, May 23, 1972.
9. Bart MJ, Macon E, Whittier FC, Baldwin RJ, Blount JH: Cadaveric kidneys for transplantation. Transplantation 31:379, 1981
10. Bart KJ, Macon E, Humphries AL, Baldwin RJ, Fitch T: Increasing the supply of cadaveric kidneys for transplantation. Transplantation 31:383, 1981
11. Prottas J, Batten HL: Health professionals and hospital administrators in organ procurement: Attitudes, reservations and their resolution. Am J Public Health 78:642, 1988
12. Prottas J: Shifting responsibilities in organ procurement: A plan for routine referral. JAMA 260:832, 1988
13. Huss AR: Transplant controversies: NFK conference takes an important step. Nephrology News and Issues 5:16, 1991
14. Roels L, Vanrenterghem Y, Waer M, Christiaens MR, Gruwez J, Michielsen P: Three years of experience with a "presumed consent" legislation in Belgium: Its impact on multi-organ donation in comparison with other European countries. Transplant Proc 23:903, 1991
15. Daar AS: Ethical issues: A middle east perspective. Transplant Proc 21:1402, 1989
16. Salahudeen AK, Woods HF, Pingle A et al: High mortality among recipients of bought living unrelated donor kidneys. Lancet 336:725, 1990
17. Nathan HM, Jarrell BE, Broznik, B et al: Estimation and characterization of the potential renal organ donor pool in Pennsylvania. Transplantation 51:148, 1991
18. US Department of Health and Human Services: Organ transplantation, issues and recommendations: Report of the task force on organ transplantation, p. 11. Washington, D.C., 1986

19. Randall T: Too few human organs for transplantation, too many in need . . . and the gap widens. JAMA 265:1223, 1991
20. Singer PA: A review of public policies to procure and distribute kidneys for transplantation. Arch Intern Med 150:523, 1990
21. Greenstein SM, Schechner R, Senitzer D, Louis P, Veith FJ, Tellis VA: Does kidney distribution based upon HLA matching discriminate against blacks? Transplant Proc 21:3874, 1989
22. Copeland JG, Emery RW, Levinson MW et al: Selection of patients for cardiac transplantation. Circulation 75:2, 1987
23. Allen *v.* Mansour: US District Court for the Eastern District of Michigan, Southern Division, 86–73429, 1986
24. Evans RW, Manninen DL, Maier A, Garrison LP, Hart LG: The quality of life of kidney and heart transplant recipients. Transplant Proc 17:1579, 1985
25. Roberts MS: Quality of life measures in liver transplantation. In Mosteller F, Falotico-Taylor J (eds): Quality of Life and Technology Assessment, p. 45. Washington, DC, National Academy Press, 1989
26. Wallwork J, Caine N: A comparison of the quality of life of cardiac transplant patients and coronary artery bypass patients before and after surgery. Quality of Life and Cardiovascular Care 1:317, 1985
27. Castelnuovo-Tadesco P: Organ transplant, body image, psychosis. Psychoanal Q 42:349, 1973

Index

Page numbers followed by (*t*) indicate tables; page numbers followed by (*f*) indicate figures.

ISBN 0-397-51172-8

90000

9 780397 511723

DATE DUE

OC 10 '97			